STEALTH GERMS
IN YOUR BODY

STEALTH GERMS
IN YOUR BODY

Erno Daniel, M.D.

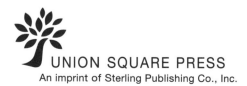

UNION SQUARE PRESS
An imprint of Sterling Publishing Co., Inc.

New York / London
www.sterlingpublishing.com

Grateful acknowledgment is made to the following: *The New England Journal of Medicine* for the excerpt by Julie Parsonnet, MD © 2005; *American Medical News* for "Infection Eyed as Culprit in Chronic Disease," © 2004.

STERLING and the distinctive Sterling logo are
registered trademarks of Sterling Publishing Co., Inc.

Library of Congress Cataloging-in-Publication Data Available

10 9 8 7 6 5 4 3 2 1

Published by Sterling Publishing Co., Inc.
387 Park Avenue South, New York, NY 10016
© 2008 by Erno Daniel
Distributed in Canada by Sterling Publishing
c/o Canadian Manda Group, 165 Dufferin Street
Toronto, Ontario, Canada M6K 3H6
Distributed in the United Kingdom by GMC Distribution Services
Castle Place, 166 High Street, Lewes, East Sussex, England BN7 1XU
Distributed in Australia by Capricorn Link (Australia) Pty. Ltd.
P.O. Box 704, Windsor, NSW 2756, Australia

Book design and layout: Scott Meola

Manufactured in the United States of America
All rights reserved

Sterling ISBN 978-1-4027-5342-8

For information about custom editions, special sales, premium and corporate purchases, please contact Sterling Special Sales Department at 800-805-5489 or specialsales@sterlingpublishing.com.

To my wife
Martha Peaslee Daniel, R.N.
and to the health of our children and their spouses
Kristina Daniel Lawson and Matthew David Lawson
Michael Peaslee Daniel and Erica Lash Daniel
Mary Daniel Gullett and Randolph Boyd Gullett
Monica Ann Daniel
and to all the family

In memory of
Ignác Fülöp Semmelweis, M.D.
1818–1865

Contents

Tables

My Inspiration

Barry J. Marshall, M.D., and J. Robin Warren, M.D.

Nobel Prize Winners in Medicine, 2005 "for their discovery of the bacterium *Helicobacter pylori* and its role in gastritis and peptic ulcer disease."

The discovery of *H. pylori* has inspired researchers to examine previous convictions with new skepticism and to pursue more aggressively the possibility of infectious causes of myriad chronic diseases, including cancers, rheumatologic diseases and atherosclerosis. . . .

In short, the clinical and scientific importance of *H. pylori* has exceeded everyone's wildest expectations. Yet the most important legacy of Marshall and Warren's award may have less to do with science than with the inspiration it should provide to medical practitioners worldwide. . . . At the time of their discovery, Warren and Marshall were physicians doing their daily jobs. . . . They had no research grants for studying ulcer disease. Rather they happened upon something interesting, and driven by curiosity, they investigated and reported it. They proved again that we, as physicians, can make ground-breaking discoveries in the course of our clinical practices if we attend to our work with open eyes, a sense of curiosity, a desire to understand, and a willingness to pursue ideas to their completion.

JULIE PARSONNET, M.D.
New England Journal of Medicine,
December 8, 2005

Author's Disclaimer

The information and descriptions presented in this book are not intended to be, nor should they be taken as, medical advice.

Information presented in this book is meant to serve as basis for discussion with your doctor, who, along with you, should make decisions about your health care.

Before considering treatment for any of the conditions described in this book, see your doctor for a proper diagnosis, even if nonprescription remedies are available.

Nor is this book intended as a comprehensive guide to the diagnosis of all possible medical conditions causing certain symptoms, but only a partial guide to some conditions that may be attributable to unsuspected infections within the body.

The information in this book does not apply to seriously ill persons with serious immune deficiencies, or those whose immune system is seriously compromised by chemotherapy or other treatments. Those persons have very special needs, and should always be in close consultation with their treating physicians and specialists.

This book is not a scientific treatise. It is a practical overview of some approaches used in the practice of day-to-day clinical medicine. It is for the use of all those who have some symptoms of concern, to enhance the likelihood of the correct identification of the cause of their condition.

1. Could It Be a Stealth Infection?

Stealth germs are infectious organisms that enter your body and can harm you, or even kill you, without you ever knowing or feeling like you had an infection.

The Story of Six Patients . . . and What They Had in Common

Millions of people worldwide carry hidden and chronic infections in their body without ever feeling like they have an infection. If they have any symptoms, those are frequently attributed to some other noninfectious condition. If left undiagnosed, such "stealth germs" can potentially harm or even kill. The goal of this book is to help you understand these stealth germs so that you can help your doctor diagnose and treat them.

Nearly everybody harbors at least one such stealth germ. If you've ever had chicken pox, or were exposed to it as a child, that virus (*Varicella zoster*) has remained alive in your system ever since. At some time during your life many of you (an estimated 20 percent of men and 30 percent of women) will develop shingles (*Herpes zoster*). This usually happens quite suddenly and is caused by the reemergence of the chicken pox virus that has been in your body since childhood. (Note: In 2006 a vaccine became available for adults, which is effective against this virus. Those of you who receive the vaccine will have some protection against developing shingles.)

My family has also been directly affected by stealth germs. In the 1970s, a close relative died of a bleeding stomach ulcer. At that time, it was not known that stomach ulcers were caused by bacteria. He had a sensitive stomach and acid indigestion for many years, but had no signs of an infection such as fever or chills. He had no other significant medical conditions and was well until he suddenly began bleeding from the ulcer. Now we know that the probable underlying cause of the ulcer and his long-standing stomach sensitivity was a low-grade infection with *Helicobacter pylori*. Might there be others like him?

To give a perspective of how such stealth infections may present themselves in many other ways, let us start with the stories of six patients. (All names have been changed, to ensure confidentiality.)

Jennifer. Jennifer, a 45-year-old woman, comes in for her regular checkup. Jennifer's case history reveals that she was born abroad and came to the United States after she was married. According to Jen's description, she has had a sensitive stomach most of her life, and it is easily irritated by even small amounts of coffee, cola, wine, or aspirin. As a result, she is careful about what she eats and drinks, and as far as she knows, she has never had an ulcer. She considers herself to be in good health, and it is unusual for her to go to the doctor. Her mother died of stomach cancer a few years earlier, and she assumes that stomach problems and stomach cancer "run in the family." She was told she has simple acid indigestion, but when treated with acid inhibitors, her symptoms continue. Is it just a hereditary sensitive stomach?

Irene. Irene, who is 55 years old, makes an appointment to be seen. She says she has recently developed rapidly progressive abdominal discomfort and unremitting diarrhea. She consulted a gastrointestinal specialist, and he performed a colonoscopy scope test. The bowel lining was inflamed, and a biopsy was sent to a pathologist, who made a diagnosis of ulcerative colitis, an incurable, noninfectious, chronic inflammatory condition of the bowel. She comes in for a general checkup, just to make sure there is nothing else going on.

Ben. Next is Ben, an 80-year-old retired man with a lifelong history of eczema over most of his body. For years he has been under the care of dermatologists, and his condition is managed with various creams and ointments. He had a tracheostomy tube placed in his neck several years earlier because of an unrelated condition. As time went on, the eczematous skin near the tube has become increasingly irritated due to moisture.

Now that area of the skin is not responding to treatment, and Ben's skin condition is getting worse. He wonders what else the doctor can suggest.

Andrea. The next patient is Andrea, a 47-year-old woman, referred to her doctor by a member of her family. Andrea has persistent, distressing pelvic discomfort. She has had these symptoms for several years, and was diagnosed with endometriosis, a gynecologic condition. She had a hysterectomy, and after her operation her recovery was slow. Since then, in addition to her persistent pelvic pains, Andrea has had a sense of malaise, and sexual intercourse has been uncomfortable. She was advised that her pains are probably due to adhesions related to the surgery, something that likely cannot be corrected. Can the doctor do anything for her?

Susan. Susan, a 67-year-old woman, goes to a new doctor for the first time. Susan has a thyroid condition. After the birth of her fifth child, she felt poorly, and was diagnosed with an underactive thyroid. Even though she was placed on a thyroid supplement, Susan never fully recovered to feeling well again. A few years later, she developed a peculiar neurological condition, with drooping and eventual atrophy of some of the muscles of one side of her face. After menopause she continued to not feel well. She felt fatigued, with achy joints, and felt cold all over her body. Susan thinks that her hypothyroidism is not being properly managed. What will her doctor think?

William. A youthful-appearing, healthy 65-year-old man with long-standing gassy stomach goes to the doctor. William has a history of acid reflux and has been on acid-inhibiting medicines for several years. The medications worked well for his acid reflux, but the chronically gassy bowels continued. His gastroenterologist told that him he had irritable bowel syndrome (IBS). His new doctor suggests he make some changes in his diet, and temporarily stop taking his various health supplements. Despite that, he continues to be gassy, and this has been interfering with his retirement. There are lots of things he cannot eat or drink, and has been told to use relaxants. Though he knows there is no cure, he thinks he will once again bring up his bowel symptoms—maybe the new doctor has some new ideas.

★   ★   ★

After meeting these patients, a doctor might think they have nothing in common. After all, one of them seems to have simple acid indigestion, the second one has an incurable inflammatory condition, the third has a chronic skin condition, the fourth adhesions from prior surgery, the fifth chronic fatigue and low-grade arthritis most likely due to her thyroid, and the last has gas from irritable bowel syndrome. Could it be possible they are all suffering from some type of stealth germ? Let us take a closer look and consider what to do next.

Jennifer. After Jennifer was examined, a blood test was ordered to check for exposure to *H. pylori*, an organism now known to cause such stomach problems. The test came back positive for prior exposure to *H. pylori*. Active *H. pylori* colonization (see Glossary) of Jennifer's gastrointestinal system was then confirmed with a stool test. She was given one week of treatment, which included two antibiotics. Her long-standing symptoms promptly resolved, and further tests showed that she no longer had active colonization with the organism. Substances that used to irritate Jennifer's "sensitive stomach" no longer do. Rather than some genetic family predisposition, it is likely that long-standing chronic inflammation of the stomach caused by carrying this same stealth germ may have predisposed her mother to develop stomach cancer.

Irene. Irene had more tests. A sample of her stool was sent to the laboratory to check for ova (see Glossary) and parasites. The test result came back showing the unusual parasitic organism *Blastocystis hominis*. *B. hominis* is considered to be nonpathogenic (see Glossary) to humans. However, even though textbooks do not generally suggest or require treatment for this presumed nonpathogen, its presence implies that this person may have come in contact with contaminated food that could also have carried other infectious organisms. She was given metronidazole, an antibiotic in pill form. Her colitis rapidly improved, then cleared completely. Subsequently she was followed for over a decade, and she had no further signs of ulcerative colitis, nor *Blastocystis* in her bowel.

Ben. How about the man with eczema? In addition to eczema, the skin near the tracheostomy had the appearance of seborrheic dermatitis, a skin condition that is also responsible for dandruff of the scalp.

Seborrheic dermatitis is often associated with the fungus *Malassezia ovale* (though this fungus may not be the only cause of the condition). Seborrheic dermatitis responds to ketoconazole (Nizoral), an antifungal available as a cream, shampoo, or pills. For this patient, ketoconazole pills were prescribed and continued for a month. During that time, not only did the dandrufflike problem near the tracheostomy tube resolve, but much of the lifelong eczema cleared from the rest of Ben's body. Followed up a couple of years later, there were no signs of relapse.

Andrea. As part of the initial evaluation, her medical history was retraced to find out when her symptoms first began. When she was a young woman, she was diagnosed with interstitial cystitis, an inflammatory condition of the bladder of unknown cause. She vaguely recalled being treated with an antibiotic and having had symptoms of pelvic infection. Though her interstitial cystitis resolved, in the years following these problems, she never quite recovered. Her pelvic symptoms would often flare up, and she was diagnosed with endometriosis. Andrea eventually underwent a surgical hysterectomy. Postoperatively she had fevers, which eventually resolved. Nevertheless, she continued to have severe pelvic pains. Further tests revealed no new abnormalities, and she was told that she had adhesions related to her surgery. Could she possibly have a smoldering low-grade stealth infection? This suspicion was heightened by minor elevation of some blood test results (Erythrocyte sedimentation rate, see page 200). The patient was given two antibiotics aimed at pelvic and bowel infections. After ten days of treatment, Andrea's symptoms improved more than 95 percent, and for the first time in several years, her general feeling of well-being also returned.

Susan. In reviewing Susan's medical history it was noted that she had received several blood transfusions due to severe hemorrhage after the birth of her fifth child. Even though this occurred decades ago, the question was now raised whether a stealth germ could have entered her system through the blood transfusion and remained there ever since. Blood tests were negative for hepatitis or other "serious infections," but showed evidence of prior exposure to an organism called cytomegalovirus. Cytomegalovirus is a member of the herpesvirus family. Some herpesviruses have been associated with palsies of the face. Susan was prescribed a commonly used antiviral medication. Within a couple of weeks, the patient began to feel markedly better. Her joint aches resolved, she no longer felt cold, and she generally felt healthy. According to Susan's husband, "the spring was back in her step." Her recovery has held up with continued use of the medication.

William. After trying numerous conventional remedies for irritable bowel syndrome, William's symptoms did not improve. Stool tests were done for ova and parasites, ulcer bacteria, and certain other bacteria, and they all came back negative. However, because some cases of so-called irritable bowel syndrome may be due to excessive bacterial overgrowth of the small intestine, William was treated with a ten-day trial course of a particular antibiotic. Within a couple of weeks, 95 percent of the patient's "irritable bowel syndrome" resolved. Later, William required one more follow-up treatment with the antibiotic. At a subsequent visit several months later, he told the doctor that he considered his long-standing "gassiness" cured.

Though different in their particulars, each of these six patients was affected by a problem common to all of them: chronic infections with smoldering stealth germs caused their persistent medical conditions. Prior to diagnosis and treatment, their symptoms were attributed to non-infectious and incurable causes. None of these patients had the classic signs of an infection such as fever or chills. As a result, during all their previous evaluations, none of them saw any reason to consult an infectious disease specialist.

If you have had a similar long-standing symptom or ailment that began suddenly at some point in your life, you have probably wondered whether it could have been caused by a contagious organism that you "caught" from someone or something. If so, you should read the rest of this book. Even if you were assured otherwise by your doctor, new medical discoveries indicate that in some cases that is indeed what may have happened.

Review Table 1 on pages 15–18. It lists conditions whose symptoms are usually not interpreted by doctors and patients as signs of infection, but which are now suspected to be caused or triggered by stealth germs.

In the past, who would have suspected that stomach ulcers were due to a smoldering bacterial infection, that cancer of the female cervix was caused by a persistent viral infection, or that childhood diabetes, multiple sclerosis, and even schizophrenia may be triggered by exposure to germs?

A Brief History of Stealth Germs

Infectious organisms should not be underestimated. In 1969 the Surgeon General of the United States declared that the "war against infectious diseases had been won," but that declaration of victory appears to have been premature. The recent assessment by Dr. Anthony S. Fauci of the National Institute of Allergy and Infectious Diseases that "the human species is in the midst of a war with the microbial world—a resilient foe that will never be completely defeated" is much closer to the mark. How slowly and insidiously some infectious organisms do their harm to human beings is just beginning to be recognized.

An important event in the history of our knowledge of infectious diseases occurred in 1847, involving Dr. Ignác Semmelweis, the Hungarian physician credited for being the pioneer in the use of hand-washing to prevent the spread of infections (for a more detailed history, see Appendix). At that time the germ theory of diseases was not known, and the deadly so-called childbed fever (puerperal fever) was killing scores of patients in hospital maternity wards. Semmelweis's friend, Dr. Kolletschka, cut his finger while at work in the hospital, and soon died of symptoms identical to those of puerperal fever. It occurred to Dr. Semmelweis that there must be some contagious factor that would explain his friend's death as well as the death of the postpartum mothers. He proposed and demonstrated that careful hand-washing by medical practitioners between treating patients could help control childbed fever. He was certain of his observation, and history has proven him right. However, his beliefs were ridiculed by his colleagues, and it was decades before his theories and methods gained wide acceptance. His story should have put us on notice.

A Personal Perspective

An event that occurred early in my career was the first step that ultimately led to the writing of this book. I was substituting for a vacationing colleague with a busy solo practice in a small community. What struck me immediately was that most of his patients were on the medicine cimetidine, commonly used in those days for treating acid indigestion and ulcers. At that time, ulcers were blamed mostly on stress, or substances toxic to the stomach lining such as aspirin, alcohol, or caffeine. However, most of his patients were not drinking excessively nor were they taking large doses of aspirin or other medicines. It puzzled me why it should be so stressful to live in that community.

It occurred to me that there was a known infectious organism called *Giardia lamblia* that lives in well water and stream water in parts of the country. When ingested, it colonizes the duodenum and causes stomach symptoms, which may continue for decades if not properly treated. At that time it was cumbersome to prove the presence of this germ by simple tests, but the organism was known to be treatable by a unique antibiotic, metronidazole. Not yet knowing about "ulcer bacteria," it seemed to me that perhaps it was *Giardia* in the local water and not stress that was causing so many in the small town to have "sensitive stomachs." Because treatment was simpler and less expensive than diagnostic testing, I treated a few of the patients with metronidazole for a week. (Note: This approach is called "empiric treatment," which is discussed in more detail in Chapter 6. See the definition of the term in the Glossary.)

Sure enough, after treatment with metronidazole, their "sensitive stomachs" improved considerably. To me, this was indirect confirmation that an infectious organism, possibly *Giardia*, was a factor in causing their symptoms. I brought it to the attention of my colleague when he returned from vacation, then thought little more about it.

A few years later, when it was reported that, rather than stress, the bacterium *Helicobacter pylori* was the cause of inflammation of the stomach (gastritis) and stomach ulcers, the lightbulb suddenly went on for me! *H. pylori*, like *Giardia*, was found to respond to the antibiotic metronidazole! Years earlier, I had unwittingly treated the organism with the right antibiotic and correctly concluded that stress was not the cause of the stomach ailment of the small-town patients I saw. Just like Semmelweis, I "knew" that it was a treatable infectious organism; I just did not know its name.

The Nobel Prize

It took several more years for the infectious cause of ulcers and gastritis to be widely accepted and fully proven. The Nobel Prize in Medicine was awarded to Barry J. Marshall, M.D., and J. Robin Warren, M.D., in 2005 for proving the connection. "Vagotomy and pyloroplasty" surgery for the treatment of ulcers, which had been popular for decades, yielded to a one-week course of antibiotics. Recently, even a single day's treatment has been shown to be effective! The number of deaths due to bleeding ulcers has decreased significantly. The year 2006 also brought the approval of a successful vaccine against cancer of the cervix, whose primary cause was found to be the infectious human papillomavirus (HPV).

Since the early 1980s I have kept my mind open to the possibility that other chronic conditions and ailments could also be caused by an unsuspected infection or infestation (see Glossary). Through more than thirty years of medical practice and over 150,000 patient encounters, I have frequently run into cases that supported my suspicions. It has become clear that many diagnoses involving "hidden" infections that may be treatable are overlooked. When making textbook diagnoses such as irritable bowel syndrome, chronic bronchitis, esophagitis, or cancer of the cervix, I have found it increasingly essential to keep asking the question: "Could an infectious organism be responsible?"

New Infections Discovered

Within the past thirty years, many conditions caused by previously unnamed, but some potentially treatable, infectious organisms have been described, including Legionnaires' disease, hepatitis C, hepatitis E, West Nile virus, and SARS (severe acute respiratory syndrome). Though some of these organisms have likely been around for a while, they came to light only when there were large enough outbreaks to focus full-scale attention. There are probably many other unsuspected, unknown, or unnamed infectious agents still remaining to be discovered and described.

While these disease-causing germs were coming to light, recognition of the body's need for its many protective "normal fellow traveler" germs has also evolved. This has led to the exploration of the benefits of so-called probiotic therapy, which attempts to aid and help restore the body's complement of "good germs," which may be disrupted or disturbed by illness or medicines.

In 2004 *The Infectious Etiology of Chronic Diseases: Defining the Relationship, Enhancing the Research, and Mitigating the Effects*, a report by the Institute of Medicine, was published. This report summarized current scientific evidence for many of our day-to-day medical observations. Because it was written for a medical and scientific audience, I felt that I should translate the science and pass it on the general public so they could understand it and apply it to their own health care. It was time to write this book.

So prepare yourself. There may be some unwelcome traveler germs in your life, which could be the cause of some of your minor annoyances or even your major medical problems. You have surely heard of herpes, hepatitis C, syphilis, and HIV/AIDS. Now prepare to meet *Giardia*, chlamydia, human papillomavirus, *Mycobacterium avium*, *Malassezia*, *Helicobacter*, *Blastocystis hominis*, and adenovirus 36. They are among the organisms detailed in the table on pages 15–18 and in an article that was published in *American Medical News*, reproduced here. Ask yourself: Could you have been exposed to, or might you be carrying, some of these organisms and not be aware of it? The answer is yes. If nothing else, you almost certainly carry the chicken pox—shingles virus. You may not know the name of some of these organisms, but could very well be intimately familiar with the symptoms they cause.

Some of these infections are treatable, some are not. Either way, you should know about them. To have a chance of ridding yourself of such organisms or to protect yourself and others against them, you need to be correctly diagnosed and properly informed. You cannot do this by yourself or by consulting the Internet. Your diagnosis will need to be individualized, taking into consideration your unique condition and circumstances, with the help of a medical professional.

That's where this book comes in. Its purpose is to provide you with the tools you can use to increase the likelihood of obtaining a correct diagnosis and appropriate treatment. It is designed to make you a truly educated consumer so you can successfully collaborate with your physician or health care provider.

Medicine is a science. Medical diagnosis and treatment are an art. This book is one diagnostician's view of the art of diagnosing conditions caused by stealth infections. To gain a full and complete perspective, it will be helpful for you to understand concepts of infection, how medical diagnoses are made, and how to participate in the diagnostic process. But first, a list of conditions and possible stealth infections that may cause them. Then read on . . . and here's to your health!

Infection Eyed as Culprit in Chronic Disease

There are skeptics, but this line of research is gaining attention.

By Susan J. Landers, *AMNews Staff*. July 19, 2004.

WASHINGTON—Imagine prescribing antibiotics for patients with atherosclerosis, or administering vaccines to prevent schizophrenia. Many researchers are thinking outside the box and are pursuing the infectious agents they believe might play a large role in causing chronic diseases.

"It is becoming increasingly acceptable and recognized that infections are probably underappreciated cause of chronic disease," said Siobhan O'Connor, MD, MPH, assistant to the director of the National Center for Infectious Diseases at the Centers for Disease Control and Prevention.

The list of chronic diseases known to be caused by infectious agents is growing. AIDS, cervical cancer, liver cancer and peptic ulcers all result from these bugs, and researchers are exploring links to heart diseases, additional cancers and psychiatric disorders. About 70% of all deaths in the United States are caused by chronic diseases, making them a prime target for research attention.

There was a time when the very idea of an infectious agent casing a chronic disease brought heaps of scorn upon the scientists who proposed it. That's what happed in the 1980s when it was suggested that ulcers were caused by *Helicobacter pylori* rather than stress and spicy food. Since then, *H. pylori* has been linked to duodenal ulcers, gastric cancer and certain types of lymphomas.

The ulcer story caused a shift in thinking that went well beyond that one disease, said E. Fuller Torrey, MD, associate director of laboratory research at the Stanley Medical Research Institute. He has been examining the role of infectious agents in schizophrenia and bipolar disorder "for more years than I care to remember." As for the current status of his research: "I wouldn't say we were respectable, but we are no longer not respectable, either."

His work with Robert H. Yolken, MD, professor pediatrics at Johns Hopkins University in Baltimore, has recently centered on the roles of the herpes viruses and a parasite, *Toxoplasma gondii*, as possible triggers for the psychiatric disorders.

But in general, even if an infection plays some role in chronic disease, it is hardly the sole cause, experts agree. Drs. Torrey and Yolken devised a working hypothesis, for instance, stating that most cases of schizophrenia are generated by infections and other environmental events occurring in genetically susceptible individuals.

The role of genes in many disorders has been recognized for about a century, Dr. Torrey noted, and the hope was that sequencing of the human genome would solve the riddle of chronic diseases and present a cure.

"If you asked someone in the mid- to late 1980s where we were going research-wise, they would say these are genetic diseases, and as soon as we get the human genome sorted out, we will identify the genes involved and we can all go home and play golf," Dr. Torrey said. "That clearly has not been the case." What is clear to him is that multiple genes are involved in many diseases, and evidence points to a link between predisposing genes and infectious agents. "That made our research of greater interest."

The role of infection in cardiovascular disease is another area that, while not yet accepted, is attracting notice, particularly since heart disease is the No. 1 killer in the United States.

For example, recent studies have linked several common infections with a person's risk of developing atherosclerosis. It is possible that a bug causes the disease, said Michael Dunne, MD, vice president of clinical development in infectious disease at Pfizer, Inc. *Chlamydia pneumoniae* is his prime suspect at the moment. "If you look at the arteries at autopsy of people with atherosclerosis, you find evidence of chlamydia in 50 percent or 60 percent of patients."

"The next step is: Can you do anything about it?" Dr. Dunne asked. That's where a series of antibiotic trials enter the picture. Although early results have not been positive, the findings from large trials scheduled for release later this summer could show whether a course of antibiotics is beneficial to heart patients.

Continuing Search for MS Trigger

The search for an infectious trigger for multiple sclerosis also has been under way for decades, said Richard T. Johnson, MD, distinguished professor of neurology, microbiology and neuroscience at Johns Hopkins School of Medicine.

When he first began researching the causes of MS in the 1960s, there was a firm conviction that the disease was due to an external agent, most likely a virus. But the early suspects turned out to result from mistakes, either misidentifications or lab contamination. That caused the idea to fall out of fashion.

Recently, however, interest peaked again. The targets are four rather ubiquitous agents: *Chlamydia pneumoniae*, herpes virus 6, Epstein-Barr virus and endogenous retroviruses. Since all are common, research is focusing on the quantity of the microbes and their location in the body. "That's very interesting but complicated argument," Dr. Johnson said.

New technologies should help with the recognition of novel agents or already established agents in chronic disease, Dr. O'Connor said. "We also need to design epidemiologic studies in a more rigorous fashion so they are reproducible," she added.

Meanwhile some of the confirmed relationships between infections and chronic disease aren't receiving sufficient consideration in the clinical world, she said. Even the well-established link between *H. pylori* and peptic ulcers may be missed.

And other established links, such as that between Lyme disease and neurologic symptoms also could go unrecognized, Dr. O'Connor said.

There are also prevention opportunities to be seized, she said. For example, physicians can tell patients that they have the power to prevent some liver cancers by avoiding exposure to the hepatitis B and C viruses.

Reprinted with permission from American Medical News, *July 19, 2004*

Table 1.
Stealth Germs and Associated Diseases

If You Have One of These Conditions Medical Diagnosis	Could It Be Due to This Particular "Stealth" Germ? Suspected or Proven Infectious Agent Causing Some Cases of the Condition
Arthritis	
Lyme disease	*Borrelia burgdorferi*
Reiter's syndrome	triggered by Salmonella typhi and other bacteria
rheumatoid arthritis	partly responsive to treatment with doxycycline
Blood Diseases	
T-cell leukemia	human T-cell lymphotropic virus type I *Strongyloides stercoralis*
AIDS	human immunodeficiency virus (HIV)
syphilis	*Treponema pallidum*
feline leukemia	feline leukemia virus
Bowel Conditions	
irritable bowel syndrome	*Giardia lamblia* *Blastocystis hominis*
persistent diarrhea post antibiotic use	*Clostridium difficile*
persistent diarrhea	bacterial overgrowth of small intestine
Brain Diseases	
dementia—multifocal encephalopathy	Creutzfeldt-Jakob prion
dementia—Whipple's disease	*Tropheryma whippelii*
dementia—kuru	prion organism
encephalomyelitis	vaccinia virus
schizophrenia	*Toxoplasma gondii*
	herpes simplex virus type 2
epilepsy	helminthic infections *Plasmodium falciparum* (malaria)
Cancer	
cancer of the stomach	*Helicobacter pylori*

cancer of the cervix	human papillomavirus
cancer of the liver	heptatitis B virus
	hepatitis C virus
cancer of the bladder (rare in US)	*Schistosoma haematobium*
cancer of colon (rare in US)	*Schistosoma mansoni*
	Schistosoma japonicum
bile ducts/cholangiocarcinoma	*Clonorchis sinensis*
	Opisthorchis viverrini
intestinal MALT lymphoma	*Helicobacter pylori*
non-Hodgkin's lymphoma	*Helicobacter pylori*
	Vibrio cholerae
	HIV
B-cell lymphoma, cutaneous	*Borrelia burgdorferi*
T-cell lymphoma	human T-lymphotropic virus
	types I and II
Burkitt's lymphoma	mononucleosis (Epstein-Barr) virus
	Plasmodium falciparum
nasopharyngeal cancer	mononucleosis (Epstein-Barr) virus
Kaposi's sarcoma	human herpesvirus type 8
mesothelioma	SV40 (Simian vacuolating virus 40)
cancer of lung in sheep	Jaagsiekte sheep retrovirus
Eye Conditions	
blepharitis	rosacea (responsive to antibiotics)
trachoma	*Chlamydia trachomatis*
Esophagus	
esophagitis (some cases)	candida
Ear	
dandruff (seborrheic dermatitis) of the ear canal	*Pityrosporum ovale*
sudden hearing loss	herpesviruses
	cytomegalovirus
Endocrine	
Type 1 diabetes	enteroviruses
thyroiditis	mumps, influenza, respiratory viruses

Fatigue	
(See also blood-borne diseases)	
persistent fatigue	hepatitis B
	hepatitis C
	herpesvirus
	cytomegalovirus
	bacterial endocarditis
syphilis	*Treponema pallidum*
Lyme disease	*Borrelia burgdorferi*
Gynecologic Problems	
menstrual cramping	pelvic infection with chlamydia
cancer of the cervix	human papillomavirus
chronic vaginitis	*Gardenella vaginalis*
	trichinella
chronic pelvic pain	pelvic infection with chlamydia, others
abdominal pain due to pelvic infection (Fitz-Hugh-Curtis syndrome)	various pelvic bacteria
Heart and Vascular	
atherosclerosis	*Chlamydia pneumoniae*
bacterial endocarditis	enterococcus
	streptococcus
	staphylococcus
Lung Conditions	
chronic bronchitis	*Mycobacterium avium*
	Chlamydia psittaci (psittacosis)
	aspergillus
asthmatic bronchitis	*Chlamydia psittaci* (psittacosis)
	respiratory syncytial virus
granulomatous spots on the lung	*Mycobacterium tuberculosis*
	Coccidioides immites
	Histoplasma capsulatum
Liver Disease	
cirrhosis	hepatitis B virus
cancer of liver	hepatitis B and C viruses
elevated liver chemistries	hepatitis B and C viruses
granulomatous "spots" on the liver	*Histoplasma capsulatum*

Nervous System Problems	
multiple sclerosis	various viruses
Bell's palsy	herpesvirus
Guillain-Barré syndrome	various organisms
Obesity	adenovirus 36
Skin Conditions	
acne	*Propionibacterium acnes*
dandruff (seborrhea)	*Pityrosporum ovale*
erythema nodosum	tuberculosis staphylococcus
erythema chronicum	Lyme disease
rosacea/ruddy cheeks	bacteria
skin cancer, nonmelanoma	human papillomavirus
hives	bacteria in the sinuses
recurrent sores	herpes simplex
skin rashes	Lyme disease, syphilis
stasis dermatitis	compounded by tinea
Stomach	
ulcers and gastritis	*Helicobacter pylori*
sensitive stomach	*Giardia lamblia*
Urinary	
chronic prostatitis	various organisms
prostate cancer	gonorrhea murine virus
Developmental Problems	
developmental problems	*Cryptosporidium* intestinal helminthic infections perinatal HIV perinatal herpesviruses Borna disease virus
congenital syphilis	*Treponema pallidum*
congenital toxoplasmosis	*Toxoplasma gondii*
congenital rubella	maternal rubella virus

Caution: Cause and effect between infectious organisms and disease is one of the most difficult things to demonstrate and prove in clinical medicine outside the animal laboratory. Only some cases—not all cases—of the above-listed conditions may be due to infection. This is only a partial list of conditions for which there is currently strong suspicion or proof. There may be many others on the list in the future, and in time some may be removed.

2. Normal Flora or Infection in the Body?

Infection and Inflammation

The question repeatedly raised in this book is whether a diagnosable infectious organism could be the cause of your present or future chronic ailment. We define stealth germs as infectious (micro)organisms that enter your body, and can harm or even kill you, without you knowing or feeling like you have an infection.

What is an infection, anyway? And what does it feel like to have one? The answer is not as simple as you might think.

An Infection by Any Other Name

The concept that germs may cause disease, or more specifically, that a specific disease is caused by a specific type of microorganism or germ in a one-to-one relationship, was not understood until 1876. This is remarkable, given the fact that the existence of microorganisms (germs) was demonstrated two hundred years earlier by Antonie van Leeuwenhoek of the Netherlands. In 1676 he observed what he called "animalcules" under a microscope he had perfected. Despite this discovery, Semmelweis in the 1850s still had a difficult time convincing even his sophisticated professional medical colleagues that contagious germs could be the cause of certain ailments.

Even now it is difficult to provide a simple definition of exactly what an infection "looks like" and "feels like," or to prove that a particular infectious organism is the sole source of someone's symptoms. Does a stomach ulcer really feel like an infection? Does early cancer of the cervix really feel like an infection? Can one infection cause more than one problem? For example, can one germ cause chronic diarrhea and at the same time progressive dementia?

Curiously, even before the formal scientific acceptance of the germ theory of disease in the 1870s, it appears that people had at least some notion of contagion or infection. In some sad chapters of history, there are known instances of deliberate "biological warfare" such as catapulting plague-infested corpses into enemy cities under siege, or giving blankets used by persons with smallpox to Native Americans.

Throughout history there have been individuals and cultures who were excellent observers of nature, such as the ancient Greeks, among them Hippocrates, the "father of medicine" and author of the well-known Hippocratic Oath (see Appendix). It would be surprising if these close observers of nature had overlooked evidence that "unclean" practices of one person could lead to the contagion of others. It is very likely that, well ahead of Semmelweis, such observant cultures may have understood intuitively that "ablution" with clean water had some role in "purification" in physical terms, not only in a spiritual sense.

Some of our everyday expressions may have derived from such observations or hunches about contagion. Words such as "pure" or "unclean" were used for many centuries to refer to persons or animals. Such terms are generally thought of as having primarily a characterological or spiritual connotation, but the context in which they were sometimes used implies a certain medical insight.

Take, for example, the concept of "unclean." "Dirt" and "filth" can be defined as any grime or foul substance which can cause physical impurity or, in other contexts, moral impurity. Most accept the commonsense notion that "dirt" that has made an object or person unclean could also potentially rub off onto something or someone else. Could it not also stick or cling to a person in some way that may affect more than appearance alone?

For example, sexually promiscuous persons in certain cultures were considered "unclean." Perhaps it is was because people noticed that after having sexual relations with a promiscuous person, something had rubbed off, which would later result in a skin rash or a genital or pelvic discharge in the previously healthy partner. Maybe "dirty old men" were labeled as such because after an intimate encounter with a promiscuous older male, a young "pure" (uninfected/uncontaminated) woman would often develop pelvic or skin maladies. In such a case "dirty" may figuratively mean "lecherous," but could also mean "contagious." Furthermore, "pure" may allude to the state of being germ free as well as spiritual purity.

Some traditional concepts about "unclean" and "unnatural" sexual practices may also indicate that past cultures had a general understanding of the natural "germ flora" of the body. Even prior to the acceptance of the germ theory, it likely did not escape observation that genital secretions could cause symptoms in the mouth when persons engaged in oral-genital contact. It would also not have escaped notice that saliva from the mouth, especially from someone who had a cold sore, could cause irritation to the pelvic or genital area. Prior to the advent of antibiotics in the late 1930s, such problems would often become persistent or even permanent.

In the case of animals, pork was and is still considered "unclean" by certain traditions and cultures. In outward cleanliness, many other mammals are not necessarily significantly "cleaner" than the pig. However, pork commonly carries trichinosis, an infection transmissible to humans and caused by the *Trichinella spiralis* organism. Before food inspection became common, this infection would spread and eventually make ill those who ate the contaminated pork. Even in this day and age there are millions of persons in the tropics who are infected by trichinosis. While many of the infected have only minor symptoms (in this way trichinosis sometimes acts as a stealth germ), heavier exposure may cause diarrhea, swelling around the eyes, sore muscles, and fever. It is possible that observers in ancient times noted that those who ate mostly pork were more likely to become ill than those who ate other kinds of meat, leading to the notion that a pig was an "unclean" animal, not just by its habits, but by some of the "dirt" it carried that could contaminate human beings.

These interpretations are mostly speculation. Nevertheless, such analysis of language and behavior can provide clues that people over the centuries may have had a commonsense understanding of contagiousness and infectious diseases prior to the establishment of scientific proof. It is now time to examine our current notions in light of the twenty-first-century understanding of infection.

What We Mean by Infection

If we are to understand stealth infections we need to clarify how an infection differs from or is related to inflammation. We also need to understand the difference between stealth germs and the harmless "health" germs, which are the normal microbial flora that cover the surfaces and parts of the inside lining of the body.

Inflammation is a protective reaction of tissue to irritation, injury, or infection, which is characterized by pain, redness, and swelling, which sometimes affects the function of the body part which is inflamed. Inflammation is not necessarily or exclusively due to infection. It can be caused by chemical irritants, such as poison oak or strong acids. Sunburn or radiation injury to various tissues and organs can also cause inflammation. Clearly, inflammation does not necessarily equal infection.

However, infections virtually always produce inflammation in the infected region. To be sure, not all infections cause *visible* inflammation, and this is why it is difficult to know by looking with the naked eye whether an infection exists or not. In some cases, only microscopic examination can detect a low-grade smoldering inflammation caused by infection in the tissues, and often there are hardly any symptoms. This is why some infections are not felt, and is also part of the reason why stealth infections were and are easily overlooked or missed. (Note: Chronic low-grade inflammation is believed to be a step in the development of cancer, as in the case of cancer of the cervix.)

Infection is generally understood to refer to the process of having germs overrun or invade a region of the body and, in the process, produce inflammation or injury to these bodily tissues, which progresses to damage or disease through a variety of biological mechanisms. But what does all this actually mean?

Where Do Infections Come From?

Most of us have a preconceived notion of what an infection is and what it feels like. However, conventional wisdom is not always right.

Most people believe that infection is the invasion of some part of the body by some foreign organism or germ that normally does not belong. They believe they "catch it" from someone else, from an animal, from eating or drinking something, from some object (such as a toilet seat), from an insect bite, or simply from droplets in the air. Such infectious germs are "pathogenic" (i.e., disease-causing), as distinguished from the normal flora of the body, which are usually harmless (see Glossary for definition of the above terms). While some of these intuitions are true, they are not completely correct. It rarely occurs to most people that the normal, domestic germ flora that covers much of our body, and is harmless in the proper location on the body, can sometimes make us sick when translocated to the wrong part of the body.

To some degree we understand this, and that is why we wash our hands after going to the bathroom. But for many, such hand washing is a cultural ritual, rather than something done based on thoughtful application of the principles of contagion control. In fact, why should one wash one's hands after urination when urine is generally sterile and free of germs? (The answer: Mostly to smell fresh. Hand washing after urination also prevents the spread of skin organisms that may colonize the genitalia or pelvic area.) Washing one's hands after cleaning up from a bowel movement has a much more important role in accomplishing contagion control, since bowel residue is often full of germs pathogenic to other areas of the body.

Do some infections in humans really not come from outside sources? Yes. In fact this is what happens when one develops a bladder infection, in which the normally sterile bladder is invaded by germs. Bladder infections are generally not caught from someone else or from a toilet seat. They are most often caused by one's own normal bowel bacteria. These bacteria travel along the skin, get near the urinary channels, make their way up the channel and overrun the bladder, an area that is normally germ-free. How can it be that when "normal" bowel bacteria enter the wrong area of the body, they cause infection, while the same bacteria in the "right" area of the body (the colon) cause no trouble and, in fact, are necessary for health? (And how is it that the bowel bacteria remain only in the colon, but rarely if ever colonize the normally germ-free small intestine directly adjacent to the colon?) One could compare this phenomenon to a bull in a china shop. It is somewhat contrary to common sense that if you put domesticated germs in the "wrong" pen, they become wild and dangerous, but if you put them back in their proper place they promptly become nondestructive again. Yet evidently this is how bacteria in the human body behave.

What Does an Infection Feel Like?

Most people think that infection happens rather suddenly and generally causes malaise, fever, inflammation, swelling, discharge at the infected site, soreness, achiness, and overall discomfort. They believe that an infection will make you feel sick and can lead to permanent harm and possibly even cause death if left untreated. And when most people think of infection, they think that it is something relatively easy to treat, usually with antibiotics, not realizing that treatment with antibiotics generally helps only bacterial and fungal infections, and does not help most viral infections. (See "antimicrobials," "antivirals," "antifungals," and "antiseptics" in the Glossary.)

But we also know from experience that not every infection results in the above scenario. Take for example the common cold. Colds usually do not cause fever, and they resolve on their own even without treatment. Bladder infections or skin boils almost never cause fever or malaise, only a feeling of local irritation.

Many acute infections are indeed characterized by prominent or even severe symptoms. (An acute infection is one that appears suddenly.) However, stealth infections are not quite what we usually think of when we think of infections. Such infections are chronic and low-grade "smoldering infections," often residing in the body for years. When the first reports appeared about the bacterial cause of ulcers, many were surprised to learn that what they thought was a "sensitive stomach" was actually a sign of an ongoing infection by the pathogenic organism *Helicobacter pylori*. This raised a number of questions. How could there be an infection when there was no fever or chills and the patient did not even feel sick? How could infection neither progress nor resolve, but cause only nonspecific symptoms for decades? How could pathogenic organisms (i.e., those that supposedly cause disease) not cause obvious disease, but merely set themselves up as a persistent local nuisance?

These issues are the reasons why it is so difficult to give simple rules for when to suspect and how to identify the presence of an infection. Doctors and patients alike do well at recognizing acute, severe infections. However, when some infections turn into chronic or smoldering conditions, most persons no longer consider their symptoms as indicative of an infection.

Do We Carry Infectious Germs Without Knowing It?

Is it possible for someone to acquire an infection with an organism that usually does not belong in the body without being aware of it or remembering any initial illness? Certainly. Such an organism could have been picked up in early childhood. Perhaps there were acute and noticeable symptoms that passed after a few days. After a while, the person may have grown accustomed to any residual symptoms (chronic gassiness, for example) as "normal" for them. There may have been even fewer symptoms if only a small number of the organisms entered the system at the time of exposure. The person may have only had a few minor or nonspecific symptoms for a brief time while the organisms gained a foothold. The connection between a few days of temporary illness, which quickly resolved, and later ongoing low-grade symptoms is never made. Being exposed to tuberculosis, or acquiring hepatitis or other infection through a blood transfusion without being aware of it are examples of such cases.

Another startling example of how some may consider symptoms of an infection to be normal, is the case of African villagers in years past who as young children were exposed to the bladder parasite *Schistosoma haematobium*, which causes schistosomiasis. *S. haematobium* causes periodic bleeding in the urine. In such villages, so many of the boys carried the parasite by the time they were teenagers that it was considered normal for young boys to have periodic bleeding, just as young girls menstruate after they reach puberty. They did not know their symptoms were due to a serious infection they carried, which would have later consequences for their health.

Curiously, a hundred years ago it was known that most adults in the United States carried *Helicobacter pylori* in their stomach. By late childhood most persons' stomach linings were colonized by these bacteria. In fact, in those days, inflammation of the stomach was so commonly found in older persons dying for other reasons that these findings and the presence of the *H. pylori* organisms were considered to be a natural consequence of aging. Now we know better. The "unexplained" decline in the incidence of stomach cancer in the United States that began after World War II curiously also coincided with the increasing use of antibiotics. Though prescribed for other infections, antibiotics likely eradicated *H. pylori* from the stomach of many carriers, which in turn led to the observed decline in stomach problems and stomach cancers in the ensuing years.

Given that similar germs are all around us and that they can hide inside our bodies for years without recognition, how do we know who is really healthy and free of contagion? How do we differentiate peculiarities of certain eras or certain regions of the world from what's "normal"? One way is to examine persons in various areas of the world who live long and healthy lives and do not have any symptoms.

What Germs Do the "Healthy" Carry?

Even completely healthy persons who are free of contagion carry germs. Our health depends critically on some of these germs. Healthy human body surfaces are ordinarily covered with innumerable bacteria and even fungi, which are referred to as the "normal flora."

What are the normal flora in the human body? Normal flora are fellow traveler "domestic animalcules" (to use the old-fashioned name given to these germs by their discoverer, Leeuwenhoek), which ride with us throughout our lives and in many ways protect us. Scientifically, when we speak of normal flora, we mean microorganisms that reside on the bodily surfaces without causing the body's defenses to mount an inflammatory reaction. These germs do not harm us, except in rare and exceptional circumstances. How is it that these germs are harmless, and are they really?

Let us examine the body's normal flora, and its role in health and disease.

The Body's Normal Flora

When looking for possible infectious organisms that could be causing symptoms of illness, we have to be able to differentiate the normal flora from infections—the "health germs" from the "stealth germs." The human body is a complex ecosystem populated by a huge number of microorganisms. Throughout our lives we live in a sea of germs, and we are covered with germs, but usually we get along with them quite well. There is no question, however, that there are certain infectious germs that can cause us harm.

Bad Germ, Good Germ

We need to learn which germs are our friends and which are our enemies. We need a "harmless list," a "most-wanted list," and finally a list of those harmful germs that can remain hidden. The "harmless" group of germs and the "most wanted" germs are found easily enough in standard infectious disease textbooks under "normal flora" and under "disease causing (pathogenic) organisms." Much of this book deals with a sub-group of disease-causing organisms, which we have chosen to call "stealth germs."

Stealth germs are infectious microorganisms that enter the body and can do you harm or even kill you. They may stay in your body for a long time and cause either minimal or no symptoms, or trigger symptoms or problems generally not interpreted by laypersons or even doctors as signs or indication of infection. (Note: This term is not used as such in the scientific medical literature.) Stealth germs are the subject of recent scientific investigations, especially in regard to their role in chronic medical conditions that until recently were attributed to something other than infectious agents. A partial list of these conditions was given in Table 1 in the first chapter.

Before we detail what is abnormal, we need to identify what germs are considered normal for the bodies of healthy human beings, in other words, which microorganisms should be placed on the "harmless list" as members of the normal flora.

Normal Flora

Our body surfaces are inhabited by a large variety of microorganisms (approximately 500 to 1,000 species and about 8,000 subspecies) that appear not to bother us by causing irritation or inflammation. Even the body of a healthy newborn (which was completely germ-free in the womb) almost immediately after birth becomes imperceptibly colonized by organisms typical of most healthy human beings. Amazingly, despite being suddenly overrun by bacteria such as staphylococcus and E. coli, most newborns show no signs of illness or inflammation. However, some other bacteria that may immediately colonize newborns may not belong to the normal flora. For this reason, nearly every infant born in the U.S. is treated with anti-infective eye drops at the time of birth, which are given to counteract possible contamination of the eyes in the birth canal by *Chlamydia trachomatis*, a common disease-causing organism. This germ frequently colonizes the female pelvic area and birth canal and may cause trachoma, which can damage the eyes and cause blindness in children. This condition is a major but preventable problem in underdeveloped countries. The ubiquity of this practice seems to suggest that even in developed countries unsuspected or undiagnosed pelvic infections in delivering mothers are common enough to warrant this intervention.

Throughout our lives, much of the human body remains overrun with bacteria and fungi. In fact, there are approximately ten times as many microorganisms on our body as there are human body cells. Body surfaces and structures such as the skin, eyes, nose, mouth, mucous membranes, outer ears, windpipe, vagina, and the large bowel all have such flora.

Other organs and areas of the body normally remain free of germs and have no normal flora at all. Such sterile areas are the bladder, lungs, small bowel, and other inner structures such as the heart, ovaries, peritoneum, liver, gallbladder, kidneys, spleen, prostate, and the inside of the eyeballs. Invasion by any microorganism, whether bacteria, virus, or fungus, of any of these normally sterile regions rapidly causes signs and symptoms of irritation, inflammation, or illness. Isn't it fascinating that the same germs that cause irritation of the bladder cause no irritation whatsoever in the bowel?

Bacteria and fungi make up the normal flora, almost exclusively. Other organisms such as viruses, mycoplasma, protozoa, and parasites are almost never found in the normal flora. In certain areas of the world, primarily in underdeveloped regions, germs such as protozoa may colonize many individuals with only minor signs or symptoms of illness or disease. That does not mean they should be considered normal flora.

How do medical scientists and biologists decide which germs on body surfaces are normal or not normal? It is not a simple process. To start, they sample, identify, and classify germs from persons from all around the world who feel healthy and who pass a basic physical. For this purpose, is it enough to accept their self-perception of health? Is it scientifically valid to classify someone as "normal" just because they say they feel well? Not quite. Some who carry stealth germs all their life (such as the chicken pox—*Varicella zoster* virus, the cause of shingles) may in fact feel perfectly well, and would pass a thorough checkup. Does that mean we should consider this virus part of the normal flora?

Furthermore, the above method is also far from foolproof, inasmuch as some germs do not grow easily in laboratory environments, only on the human body. They may be missed during attempts to sample and collect the flora of body surfaces. Nevertheless, over time, the basic list of the germs commonly found on normal healthy human beings has become known. A partial list is provided in Table 3 and Table 4 below.

A fascinating characteristic of the normal resident flora is that when these bacterial or fungal colonies on our bodies are disturbed, they quickly reestablish themselves in just the right numbers. Transient flora may colonize the body for brief periods of time without doing apparent harm but do not take up permanent residence. However, the normal flora almost always returns to its usual numbers and proportions.

To more precisely define the status of fellow-traveler organisms on our body, relationships are described and labeled in textbooks of biology and medicine as "symbiotic" or "parasitic." A symbiotic relationship is understood to describe a persistent, close association between two different organisms whereby the relationship benefits both. In our case, this would apply to the association between a human or animal and one or more type of germs. A parasitic relationship usually indicates a relationship whereby groups of organisms, such as germs, are harbored by the host while contributing nothing and even being potentially damaging to the survival and health of the host.

The Protective Role of Normal Flora

Germs of the normal flora are not only harmless but in fact play an important role in protecting us and keeping us healthy. For example, one function of the bacteria on the surfaces of the body is to continually stimulate and probe the immune system by continued generation of certain levels of immunoglobulins M and G and certain lymphocytes. Additionally, because of their sheer number, germs of the normal flora crowd out disease-causing germs and prevent them from gaining a foothold or multiplying sufficiently to cause irritation or disease.

Another example is the helpful role of the normal germs that cover the vaginal area. These bacteria (among them lactobacillus) make lactic acid, which creates an acidic condition and makes the local environment unfavorable to other invading bacteria. Bacteria in our large bowel and colon (there are upwards of a hundred trillion of them) also play a beneficial role by promoting the digestion and fermentation of foods not fully absorbed in the small intestine. By this process, the intestinal bacteria produce vitamin K and several B vitamins. Poorly nourished persons treated with prolonged courses of antibiotics often suffer vitamin deficiencies due to suppression of these vitamin-producing bacteria. (Note: This is also the reason why persons treated with the anticoagulant warfarin are advised to avoid certain fibrous vegetables whose residue in the bowel enhances production of vitamin K by bowel bacteria, which in turn partly cancels the benefit of warfarin.)

Even on abnormal surfaces of the body, such as open wounds, certain bacterial colonies are necessary and help to promote proper wound healing. Despite the conventional wisdom, trying to keep a wound sterile is generally not a good idea. Clean, yes, but sterile, no. Have you ever wondered how an open sore such as an anal fissure ever heals, despite the fact that it is constantly contaminated by bowel material? Remarkably, it does, despite the constant "contamination." If you scrape yourself or bite your tongue, the wound won't be sterile. Yet it heals. Dogs lick their wounds, and by doing so they introduce mouth bacteria into the wound, yet most of their wounds heal without medication. Dog bites can cause serious infections in humans, yet how is it that a dog chewing on its wound doesn't cause it to become seriously infected? Perhaps, for dogs, licking a wound cleans it without sterilizing it. Biology is truly remarkable.

There is also accumulating evidence that infants and younger children benefit from exposure to a varied group of microbes. If the infant's immune system receives only limited exposure, it may not develop to work as well as it should. There is preliminary evidence that children who have been exposed to very small doses of even potentially disease-causing germs alongside their normal flora may be less likely to develop allergies and asthma in later years compared with those meticulously protected against all infectious exposure. This does not mean that you should deliberately expose your child to harmful germs! However, raising a child in an excessively sterile environment may be counterproductive. So what is the happy medium? Unfortunately, no specific recipe exists beyond simple common sense.

Different Germs in Different Areas of the Body

Germ distribution is not uniform throughout the body. In fact, different parts of the body have different normal flora, influenced through a process called host tropism. Not only are there different organisms on different body surfaces, but there may be a different balance of the organisms, i.e., a different relative distribution, on different body surfaces. This distribution may further vary in the young vs. the old, or in healthy vs. unhealthy individuals.

The yeast monilia (*Candida albicans*) is a good example of this issue of proportion and balance. There is always some yeast on the body surfaces, and, if present in the right amount, there will be no irritation or inflammation. However, if antibacterial antibiotics are taken and the normal bacterial flora is suppressed, the balance may be disturbed, and the yeast can proliferate on a particular surface (often the vaginal area, mouth, throat, or regions of the skin). This "overgrowth" can cause irritation, usually called a yeast infection. We generally do not catch a yeast infection from someone else. An element of our own normal germ layer simply multiplies out of control when some other members of the protective veneer are overwhelmed.

The case of yeast infection is one example of how even beneficial normal flora can occasionally turn on us. But we need to be cautious about overdiagnosing yeast infections. There are some erroneous ideas about the cause-and-effect relationship between the presence of candida and its role in producing various ailments. Its mere presence is harmless and normal. It is its disproportionate overgrowth that is of concern. Precisely what proportion of yeast to bacteria constitutes a problematic yeast infection? There is no hard and fast rule. This is one of the difficulties in determining whether colonization of some part of the body with an organism is truly normal, or the cause of some local nuisance. Most often it is a matter of judgment based on observation, rather than subject to quantitative analysis.

We Are Not Uniform

As you can see, it is difficult to precisely define and delineate the normal germ flora, and determine its correct distribution in a healthy body as opposed to one with disease. Furthermore, the normal human flora may not be the same over the course of one's life. For example, normal flora is influenced by hormones and hormonal changes, which is why, for example, teenagers develop acne, and older people generally do not. Also, vaginal flora in young girls before the onset of puberty is different than that in women of childbearing age and in those who are postmenopausal.

In addition to predictable age differences, there may also be individual differences. There is growing evidence that microbial flora is rather unique in each healthy individual, almost to the degree that you can think of it as a "microbial fingerprint." There are variations related to diet, such as when teenagers break out with acne after they eat certain foods. There are also dissimilarities in the normal flora of different ethnic groups, or in persons with chronic conditions such as diabetes. Additionally, we can't really say what is normal for someone who lacks a chemical called secretory IgA (immunoglobulin A), which is part of our surface-protecting immune system. One in six hundred otherwise normal persons have this deficiency. Is their normal flora different from those who do not have this deficiency? Should this change our judgment about what is normal or abnormal for them? Only limited specific information is available to answer such questions; in treating patients such differences are essentially impossible to document or quantify.

Normal Flora on the Rampage

As we keep discovering, in addition to known pathogens, even our own normally harmless "health germs" can cause disease. This occurs not only when the relative balance is off, but when these germs enter the wrong area of the body. Take for example E. coli (*Escherichia coli*, named for the German bacteriologist Dr. Theodor Escherich). Our large bowel is inhabited by literally trillions of these bacteria. They usually cause no problem, unless they migrate to the bladder. There they cause an excessive inflammatory response, which is commonly labeled a bladder infection. In the gut of healthy individuals, these and other colon bacteria generally confine themselves to the large bowel, and under normal conditions almost never enter or colonize the neighboring small intestine, though the passage between the two is open. If these organisms do enter the small bowel and grow in significant numbers, diarrhea, gassiness, and other gastrointestinal symptoms can result.

Our skin is full of "staph" organisms (*Staphylococcus aureus*), which are ordinarily harmless. However, if staph bacteria invade the nasal passages, they can be the source of a chronic low-grade irritation, and even spread to the blood and seed distant infections in the body such as infectious osteomyelitis or endocarditis. Certain strains of staph can cause boils on the skin, or impetigo. Additionally, if normal skin germs are introduced into the bursa of the elbow, a normally sterile bodily fluid, they will cause septic bursitis.

Mouth bacteria cause no problem when they stay in the mouth. Even if we bite the inside of our cheek, the wound generally heals without antibiotics. However, if we accidentally bite elsewhere through the skin into the flesh, the bite wound usually develops a serious infection. When allowed to proliferate excessively because of poor dental hygiene, germs normally found around the gums have been implicated in causing cardiovascular and kidney diseases.

How can the same organisms be innocuous and a source of dangerous infection, simply depending on location and their numbers? Such are the mysteries that make it difficult to provide a simple definition for an infection. If all of this sounds a bit complicated, it is. Nevertheless, there are ways to make sense of it all and make reasonable judgments about when treatment is needed or not needed.

Who Is "Normal"?

As a broad generalization, if we feel well day after day, we are generally considered healthy. However, trying to make an objective determination of who has normal flora based solely on whether that individual feels healthy or not poses difficulties. Asymptomatic carriers, who do not have apparent symptoms, may harbor pathogenic microorganisms yet actually feel quite well. Conversely, just feeling poorly by itself–such as after some serious personal loss, or subsequent to a brain injury–does not mean that one is truly ill or carries a pathologic germ, a disease, or an infection.

Why does this even matter? What about those who carry stealth germs? If they feel reasonably well, aren't they basically healthy? Just because their bodies harbor a germ that's not on the normal flora list, are they really at risk for certain problems? This is an excellent question, which requires further examination of cause-and-effect issues between germs and illnesses.

However, before delving into further details of stealth infections, let us briefly examine some recent concepts about measures that may help the maintenance (and feeding and watering) of our magnificent and beneficent normal flora.

The tables on the next page list those regions of the body that are sterile and the normal flora of the human body.

Table 2.
Germ-free Regions/Tissues in the Human Body

Brain

Blood

Liver

Spleen

Kidney

Bladder

Lower bronchi and alveoli

Table 3.
Normal Flora in the Human Body

Microorganisms	Region of the Body
Bacteroides species	colon, throat, vagina
Candida albicans	mouth, colon, vagina
Clostridium species	colon
Corynebacterium species (diphtheroids)	nasopharynx, skin, vagina
E.coli and other coliforms	colon, vagina, outer urethra
Gardenella vaginalis	vagina
Haemophilus species	nasopharynx, conjunctivae
Lactobacillus species	mouth, colon, vagina
Neisseria species	mouth, nasopharynx
Pseudomonas aeruginosa	colon, skin
Staphylococcus aureus	nose, skin
Staphylococcus epidermitis	skin, nose, mouth, vagina, urethra
Streptococcus faecalis (enterococcus)	colon
Viridans streptococci	mouth, nasopharynx

Table 4. Medically Important Organisms of the Normal Flora		
Location	**Important Organisms**	**Less Important Organisms**
Skin	*Staphylococcus epidermitis*	*Staphylococcus aureus*, *Corynebacterium* (diphtheroids), various streptococci, *Pseudomonas aeruginosa*, anaerobes (such as *Peptostreptococcus*), yeasts (such as *Candida albicans*)
Nose	*Staphylococcus aureus*	*Staphylococcus epidermitis*, *Corynebacterium* (diphtheroids), various streptococci
Mouth	Viridans streptococci	various streptococci
Dental plaque	*Streptococcus mutans*	
Gums	various anaerobes, such as *Bacteroides*, *Fusobacterium*, streptococci, actinomyces	
Throat	Viridans streptococci	various streptococci including *Streptococcus pyogenes* and *Streptoccus pneumoniae*, *Neisseria* species, *Haemophilus influenzae*, *Staphylococcus epidermitis*
Colon	*Escherichia coli* (coliforms), *Bacteroides fragilis*	bifidobacteria, eubacterium, *Fusobacterium*, lactobacillus, various aerobic gram-negative rods, *Streptococcus faecalis* and other streptococci, *Clostridium perfringens*
Vagina	lactobacillus, E. coli, group B streptococci	various streptococci, various gram-negative rods, *Bacteroides fragilis*, *Corynebacterium* (diphtheroids), *Candida albicans*
Urethra		*Staphylococcus epidermitis*, *Corynebacterium* (diphtheroids), various streptococci, various gram-negative rods, *Mycobacterium smegmatis*

Protecting Normal Flora: The Role of Probiotics

Is there anything we can do to help improve upon the amazingly complex and nearly miraculous workings of the human body and its microbial cover? There just may be.

One of the fascinating features of the body's normal flora is that it maintains itself without any deliberate effort or intervention. The human body does very well in keeping itself fully functional and in equilibrium without outside intervention, unless it is significantly injured by physical, chemical, or biological insults or hampered by inborn or acquired malfunctions. All we usually need to do is feed and water it, periodically rinse its surface, and it usually takes care of the rest. The body will do so for many decades, even if we feed it junk food and ingest liquids of questionable purity or nutritional value. Clearly some dietary regimens are healthier than others, but the body still mostly self-maintains despite what we do to it.

The Remarkable Body

In a healthy person, most of the time the body keeps reestablishing its own equilibrium of normal fellow traveler germs, regardless of whether we wash our hands frequently, bathe or shower regularly, use deodorants and antibacterial soaps, injure our skin or other surfaces, take antacids or laxatives, and even if we take antibiotics. On occasion, if we are ill or take certain medicines, restoration of the normal balance of the flora may not occur so readily, rapidly, or automatically, even if we are otherwise healthy. Moreover, in seriously ill persons, such as those with immune deficiencies due to advanced AIDS or chemotherapy, more severe problems can occur with the germ cover. Pathogenic organisms may overrun the surfaces of the body and the normal flora is not able reestablish itself. Management of these severe conditions is beyond the scope of this book and should be entrusted to specialist physicians who deal with serious illnesses.

Antibiotics and the Body's Flora

In otherwise healthy individuals, it is most often treatment with antibiotics that causes the normal bacterial flora in certain regions of the body to be thrown into disarray. Why the bacterial flora? And what exactly is an antibiotic? The term is used somewhat loosely by the public and sometimes even in the medical community.

Some use the word "antibiotic" to refer to medicines that "kill" germs in general, though others hold the impression that antibiotics are used mostly against bacteria specifically. Various definitions abound. All agree that antibiotics are widely used in the prevention or treatment of infectious diseases. Generally antibiotics are defined as drugs used to treat infections caused by bacteria and microorganisms.

We should try to use more precise medical terms. Antimicrobial should be the general term for "germ-killer." Antibacterial should be used for antimicrobials that treat bacteria. The term "antiviral" is already the term most often used to refer to antimicrobials aimed at eradicating viruses, and the term "antifungal" is generally used to indicate substances used to eradicate fungal organisms. Using more precise terminology helps minimize confusion, and helps us understand why commonly used antibiotics suppress primarily bacteria.

Normal Flora Out of Equilibrium

A classic example of a loss of equilibrium of the body's normal germ cover is the pelvic yeast infection that some women develop when taking antibiotics. (More precisely, antibacterials, as opposed to antivirals or antifungals. The latter actually treat yeast infections.) A pelvic yeast infection is characterized by itching, burning, and white-colored vaginal discharge. This condition is due to the overgrowth of one's own resident Candida albicans fungus, which may overgrow exuberantly when the naturally occurring bacteria are suppressed.

Remarkably, soon after antibacterial antibiotics are stopped, even without specific treatment, such yeast infections usually recede, and the body's surfaces reestablish their former balance of germs. However, it is also true that taking measures to suppress the excess yeast (with an antifungal or use of probiotics) can help to more rapidly restore the normal balance of the flora.

When taking antibacterial antibiotics, alteration of the normal bowel flora can also occur, leading to gastrointestinal symptoms such as bloating and diarrhea. Ordinarily, colonies of bacteria in the bowel are undergoing constant change. Large numbers are passed out of the body daily. When taking antibiotics, the population changes even more. When too many of the organisms of the normal bowel flora are suppressed, the bowel may be overrun by one's own *Clostridium difficile* bacteria, which also produces a diarrhea-causing toxin. In such a case the patient will usually feel ill, with significant diarrhea, and sometimes will run a fever. Taking certain medicines to help suppress the activity of *C. difficile* and reestablish the normal flora in the bowel will hasten recovery. Taking some preventive steps, such as taking ingestible preparations of probiotics, may reduce the chance of this happening in the first place.

What Are Probiotics?

In recent years, increasing attention has been focused on measures that may aid the maintenance and hasten the restoration of normal flora in parts of the body where such flora has been disturbed by illness or medications. Probiotics were defined in a 2001 report from the World Health Organization as "live microorganisms which, when administered in adequate amount, confer a health benefit on the host." The probiotic organisms used in treating persons are generally not part of the normal human flora, but their close relatives. Prebiotics are generally understood to be foods which have ingredients that do not digest fully, but which pass through the intestines to the colon, where they produce a beneficial effect by providing nutrients which promote the growth of some of the logcal resident "beneficent" bowel bacteria, such as bifidobacteria.

The concept of pro- and prebiotics is not new. As noted earlier, cultural and language traditions indicate that even in antiquity people made observations that showed insight into medical and bodily processes. Before antibiotics, soured milk was used as "medicine." Fermentation has been used for centuries as a method for preserving foods. Biblical passages mention the use of cultured dairy products. Presently, the use of probiotics in medical treatment is being reevaluated with twenty-first-century scientific methods.

How Do Probiotics Work?

Microbes used as probiotics are not members of the normal flora of the body, but instead are a group of nonpathogenic live microorganisms of low virulence. Some of the best-studied organisms are bacteria of the *Lactobacillus* and *Bifidobacterium* species. We will discuss them and exactly how they do their work in greater detail in chapter 7.

The evidence is that probiotics assist the normal flora damaged by disease or medicines. They do this in part by substituting for the healthy flora. They appear to work by outcompeting pathogenic organisms for the nutrients that the pathogens need to grow. There is also evidence that probiotic microorganisms can modify toxins produced by pathogens, or modify toxin receptors found in the gut wall. They may also help stimulate immune responses to pathogens. Researchers are currently investigating these mechanisms in detail.

Regardless of the precise details of how they work, probiotics have been shown in outcome studies to help the body overcome infections of mucosal surfaces, such as the gut (where they are most useful), the vagina (where they may protect against yeast infection), and the respiratory tract. Their benefit has been reproducibly shown in diarrheal illnesses, especially those of children, and especially in those diarrheal conditions related to the use of antibacterial antibiotics.

When undertaking medical intervention or treatment, not only should there be no harm, but there should be measureable benefit from the intervention. Thus, as one investigates and considers the role of probiotics in restoring or maintaining healthy body functions, it will not be enough to use them merely because they may contain certain colonies of natural organisms that are supposed to be "good for you." Their use should be based on more than just the observation that persons who take them feel better. The true health benefits of such therapy should be demonstrated in ways that constitute acceptable scientific proof.

The Call for Careful Scientific Inquiry

Even without treatment with probiotics, many conditions that result from disturbances in the equilibrium of the normal flora are handled by the body itself in otherwise healthy individuals. However, research is underway to document the extent and degree of benefit of probiotics in preventing traveler's diarrhea, respiratory infections in children, dental cavities, inflammatory bowel disease, intestinal inflammation in patients with cystic fibrosis, irritable bowel syndrome, and *Clostridium difficile* bowel infections. There is also some early evidence that probiotics may delay the onset of certain types of diabetes and that they strengthen the weakening immune systems of the elderly. There is some evidence of benefit in reducing absences due to illness of otherwise healthy infants in day care centers and healthy adults in the workplace.

Scientific principles are straightforward, but real-life individuals are complex. One needs to be careful to avoid broadly generalizing results of an isolated study to all persons with various conditions, a mistake frequently made. The International Scientific Association for Probiotics and Prebiotics was formed in 2000 to provide a forum for serious scientific discussion of the results of studies in this field.

There should also be caution about assuming that all probiotics are of equal benefit. If commercially available preparations of probiotics are prepared carelessly, they themselves may contain unwanted pathogens. Adverse effects are observed in approximately 1 percent of persons taking probiotics.

Despite all of these cautions and considerations, probiotic "health germs" are being increasingly shown to have a role in protecting health by helping to maintain and restore normal flora, especially when the normal flora has been disturbed. A good case can be made for taking probiotics when one takes antibiotics. We will return to this important topic in much more detail once again in chapter 7 when considering the treatment of infections.

But what does all this have to do with stealth germs? To understand them and how they affect us, we had to set the foundation of knowledge about how microorganisms, whether harmless or harmful, behave and interact in the body. Just as in math, we needed to learn addition and subtraction before we do algebra. Now we are ready to move on to stealth infections and their diagnosis.

Germs That Do Not Belong in Your Body

Now that we have some perspective on the normal germ flora of our body and how it maintains itself, let us examine what happens when organisms other than the ones that belong to our beneficent normal flora gain a foothold on your body. How do we catch these germs? Do they necessarily cause harm? Conventional wisdom suggests that carrying germs that are not part of the normal flora is generally not good for you.

Some invaders arrive in moderate numbers but die off rapidly without being able to gain a foothold on the particular surface where they landed due to inhospitable conditions, such as temperature, acidity, or lack of moisture. Other invaders do their best to overrun the body but run into its defenses. A great majority of the time, without any outside help or assistance, the body's immune system repels attempted invasions by germs. If you catch a cold, it usually resolves. If you have a small boil, it heals. Even some cases of pneumonia and tuberculosis eventually clear up without treatment with antimicrobials or antibiotics.

Other germs that land are rapidly placed in check by the body's immune defenses, but they are only partly neutralized and are able to "hang on" and hide in moderate numbers in some nook or cranny of the body. They may establish a small colony somewhere and live quietly, bringing only minimum attention to themselves, waiting for a later opportunity to proliferate. They become stealth germs.

Take the case of cold sores. If you have a cold sore, it appears to go away by itself. However, at some later time it may reappear without re-exposure to someone else with the condition. Clearly, once it had landed, the herpes simplex virus, which causes cold sores, gained a foothold and remained in your system, noticed or unnoticed. It periodically re-emerges to the surface. The *Varicella zoster* virus, which causes the well-known childhood illness chicken pox, often hides for decades before it re-emerges as shingles. How does our immune system deal with these and other infectious organisms? And why does our immune system not always get rid of them successfully?

The Remarkable Immune System

Starting early in life, a person's immune system develops a remarkable "memory" for infections. It develops specific antidotes—called "antibodies" in the form of immune globulins—against infectious organisms it encounters. It stockpiles cells that make these antibodies in locations such as the bone marrow, spleen, lymph nodes, tonsils, and appendix. This mechanism of the body's own native immunity creates a rapid response when confronted with less than overwhelming numbers of previously encountered invaders.

Much of the building and maintenance of this native immunity occurs naturally and imperceptibly, every single day of our lives. In fact, encountering small numbers of various germs is necessary to build and maintain such responses and such stockpiles. One example of how remarkably this works is what happens to infants, who reside in a germ-free womb until birth. Upon birth they are immediately exposed to the sea of germs all of us live in. The mother's preformed antibodies, which the infant receives from the maternal blood via the placenta, protect the infant almost fully against the billions of germs they are exposed to. However, protection from these preformed antibodies lasts for only a few weeks. By then the infant's own immune system is successfully gearing up its defenses against the normal flora of their environment. In the meanwhile, further protection is obtained from antibodies in the colostrum which the baby ingests during breastfeeding.

The process of vaccination was developed to enhance the natural process of building immunity in children as well as adults. Vaccines artificially expose us to small numbers or small parts of certain germs, or less virulent cousins of particular disease-causing organisms. This exposure helps to stimulate our immunity and create antibodies against particular diseases. When the immune system is geared up this way, then we suffer little or no ill effects if we encounter pathogenic germs in moderate numbers. Trouble may arise when there is exposure to overwhelming numbers of known germs, or exposure to previously unencountered germs in large numbers. How much exposure is moderate, large, or over-whelming? There is no generally accepted amount. We need to consider the concept of virulence, a term that is formally defined below.

Generally, most of us are able to recognize when some invading infectious organism seriously affects us. We experience fever, chills, cough, pain, drainage, swelling, inflammation, and so on. In such cases, we expect that either the infection will resolve, or we will be given some medicines that will clear up the infection.

Most of us also believe that most, if not all, infections are curable. While this is generally true for bacteria and fungi, it is not as well known that doctors have virtually no weapons against viruses. Consider that there is no specific medication that can cure severe acute respiratory syndrome (SARS), bird flu, Ebola virus, or even AIDS. This also true for the vast majority of other viral illnesses—they are neither curable nor even treatable with medicines. For example, medicines used to treat influenza do not truly cure the illness nor kill and fully eradicate the virus. Antiviral medications exist against fewer than a dozen of the thousands of viruses that infect human beings, and essentially none of them are curative. For the most part, either the body's own immunity takes care of viral infections or else it does not.

Even in the case of bacteria, some of the numerous antibacterial antibiotics do not actually kill the bacteria. Certain antibiotics, such as sulfa, merely prevent bacteria from multiplying further, and are considered to be bacteriostatic. In the presence of such medicines, the body relies on its own immune system to mop up the invading bacteria that are already present, while the antibiotic holds the proliferating invasion at bay. This is one reason why patients with a seriously malfunctioning immune system, such as those with AIDS, may still die of a bacterial infection, despite being treated with the best available antibacterial antibiotics. Only some of the antibiotics are truly germ killers, or what biologists call bactericidal.

Even a normally functioning immune system, with or without the help of antimicrobials, cannot always kill every last invading germ. Some of these germs can be very clever at hiding out. Tuberculosis organisms may hide for decades in a few lymph nodes in the body. Herpesviruses hide in nerve roots, only to re-emerge periodically when the opportunity arises and the body's defenses are distracted. The fungal spores of *Coccidioides immites*, which cause coccidioidomycosis (valley fever), may remain dormant in the lungs or the spleen in clusters called granulomas. Other germs, such as the hepatitis C virus, keep circulating, held partly in check by the body's immunity so that they do not multiply enough to produce overt signs of illness. Without spreading further, *Helicobacter pylori* germs remain localized on the lining of the stomach, and *Giardia lamblia* continues to reside on the surface of the duodenum. Human papillomavirus continues to colonize the surface of the cervix, and chlamydia colonies may remain in the cervical canal and the fallopian tubes on in the walls of blood vessels. These germs continue to stay alive and may gradually cause some degree of tissue damage. In such cases, are we infected and contagious to others, or are we simply "carriers" of these germs?

Defining Our Terms

To be sure that we use words correctly and meaningfully in talking about infections, let us define some terms.

Infection. Infection is generally understood to refer to a disease condition caused by germs that are spread or communicated in any matter. ("Contagion" is a term that applies more concisely to spread of infection in a way that requires personal contact with the infected person.) All infections are infectious but only some are considered contagious. For example, bladder infections are not contagious; they generally cannot be passed on to someone else. Influenza is infectious and is transmitted through droplets in the air, but it does not require direct person-to-person contact. Sexually transmitted diseases are generally contagious, requiring personal contact; they are not transmitted to others by sneezing in a roomful of people, though a few might be passed on by touching contaminated objects. Unfortunately there is no simple rule that can be given for all germs; we need to understand each of them individually.

Pathogen. A germ or microorganism capable of causing disease is called a pathogen. Some germs cause disease in animals or plants, but are not pathogenic to human beings. Some of our own normal flora is pathogenic under certain circumstances, or in certain regions of the body and ogenic under certain circumstances, or in certain regions of the body and not others, as discussed above.

Virulence. This term describes how powerful a particular disease-causing germ is, in terms of how many of the organisms are required to cause harm. Scientists measure a germ's virulence in two ways. The number of organisms required to kill half of the hosts is known as LD50—lethal dose 50 percent. How likely the germ is to make you sick is measured by the number needed to cause an infection in half of the hosts, ID50—infectious dose 50 percent. Even the same species of germ can have more or less virulent varieties, called strains. The influenza virus has more or less virulent strains, which may change from year to year. Cholera also has more virulent and less virulent forms, as do E. coli and staphylococcus. Finally, in some persons with weaker immunity the same infection may be more virulent than in those with normal immunity.

Opportunistic Infection. Opportunistic organisms are those that rarely if ever cause disease in persons with normal immune systems, but can cause serious infections in patients whose immunity is compromised due to various illnesses, cancer chemotherapy, or AIDS. Some of these opportunists are members of the normal flora of the body. Under normal circumstances they remain under control in modest numbers on the body's surfaces that they usually inhabit, but given the right conditions, they will overrun undefended territory.

If We Carry Germs, Are We Infected?

If we persistently carry germs that don't belong to the normal flora, are we considered to be infected? Yes. However, the terms "colonized" or being a "carrier" are also often used, so it is useful to designate them separately, though the definitions and meanings overlap.

Colonization. When an organism that is not part of the normal flora of the body establishes an ongoing presence, the person is said to be colonized by that organism. At times we can have such colonization (or infestation, though this term more often refers to insects such as lice) of a part of our body with very little evidence of active infection. There is no noticeable inflammatory response by the colonized tissues of the body. For example, after touching patients infected with antibiotic-resistant staph (MRSA, or methicillin-resistant *Staphylococcus aureus*), the skin of health care workers can become temporarily colonized with this particular hazardous strain of the bacteria. While it causes no irritation to the skin of the carrier (see below), it can be passed on to infect others who may have heightened susceptibility to infections.

Carrier State. In a sense we are all carriers of microorganisms. However, in medical parlance, a carrier is someone who harbors a potential pathogen and therefore can be the source of infection to others. "Asymptomatic carrier" describes a person who has no outward signs or symptoms of an infection (visible inflammation, for example), yet carries a pathogenic organism, which may be shed and passed on to others. Sexually transmitted diseases are the most notorious infections in this category. After exposure, some persons may carry the syphilis bacteria for decades, and for extended periods of time they do not feel sick and have minimal obvious signs of illness. However, the organism is present in their blood and bodily fluids and may be contagious to others. Some women carry colonies of chlamydia in their vaginal area. They have minimal symptoms, yet may transmit the germ to the eyes of their infant at childbirth, or to others through intimate contact.

Contagion/Contagious. This term generally refers specifically to disease transmission by direct or partially direct contact. Someone who is contagious is capable of transmitting disease-causing germs to others.

The Status of Stealth Germs

Stealth infections in the body are generally characterized by carrier state and colonization. How do we become colonized, and how do we become carriers? By being exposed to pathogenic organisms through contact with contaminated individuals, foods, materials, or biological substances. The strength of our own immune system, as well as the virulence of the organism encountered, determine the likelihood of becoming infected. Less-virulent germs require close contact with someone or something harboring large numbers of the germs, while highly virulent respiratory germs such as tuberculosis can be "caught" even if small numbers are transmitted over some distance by droplets in the air. Transmission methods for some organisms remain a mystery. For example, we are still not clear about how people catch *Helicobacter pylori*. There is suspicion but no proof that contaminated food or water is the source.

What if we don't remember such a contact, or becoming infected? This often happens. Some germs may cause only minor, transient symptoms when they first arrive in moderate numbers. As the immune system fights back, the person rapidly feels better and concludes that they "got over it, whatever it was." For example, someone who acquires a germ after a blood transfusion may temporarily feel a bit feverish a few days later but chalk it up to a minor "transfusion reaction."

Germs may sneak into the system in such small numbers or in a hidden area such as the female pelvis that they produce very little in the way of a noticeable inflammatory reaction. Such infections are called subclinical infections. Yet despite the minimal or hidden initial disturbance, such germs still gain a foothold and remain in the body. As an example, on routine testing, persons may be found to have an abnormal (positive) reaction to a tuberculosis (TB) skin test without ever being aware of being sick or remembering exposure to someone with TB. Nevertheless, the positive test is sign that the organism has truly entered the individual's system. Only prolonged antimicrobial (antituberculous) treatment will eradicate the tuberculosis germ from its hiding place.

Susceptibility Varies from Individual to Individual
Who becomes colonized and who doesn't? Is everyone equally susceptible? Clearly not. Some persons truly have the proverbial iron constitution. They never seem to catch anything and they never seem to get sick. (There are very rare persons who are even resistant to catching HIV/AIDS despite repeated exposure. Such persons have been found to have an inborn protection provided by the CCR5-Δ32 deletion in one of their chromosomes.) Other people appear to become infected much more readily, and in some cases we know why. For example, patients with Type 1 or Type 2 diabetes are at increased risk for urinary, lower respiratory tract, and other common infections, such as yeast infection. It is also

known that *Giardia lamblia* is more likely to colonize the duodenum of those who are born with a deficiency of secretory IgA (immunoglobulin A) in the lining of their stomach. Similar variations in immunity may determine why some persons have recurrence of their herpes simplex eruption almost every month, and others only very rarely, if at all. An interesting feature of stealth germs is that those carrying one of these organisms are often more likely to develop a serious reaction when exposed to a new one. More about this later.

Regardless of whether it happens noticeably or not, a large number of persons wind up with stealth germs in or on their body. How can we prove beyond a shadow of a doubt whether such a germ is causing current symptoms or whether it may cause problems that become evident later, such as certain cancers? The answer is not straightforward, and perhaps that is why cause-and-effect relationships between stealth germs and chronic conditions are only now being clarified, despite the acceptance of the germ theory of diseases for over 130 years, and the existence of antibiotics and antimicrobials for the past seventy years.

After reading and understanding all of this material, you might be wondering whether certain symptoms you have could be due to a stealth infection. Even if your suspicion is correct, you will need some diagnostic proof if there is to be treatment or management. You cannot do this by yourself. Even health care professionals occasionally overlook stealth germs as the underlying culprit in various chronic conditions.

Factors that hamper the diagnosis of smoldering infections are lack of awareness of the concept of stealth germs, variations in individual reaction to infection, as well as the complexities of physician–patient communication about multiple vague and nonspecific symptoms.

To see how we can make the complicated diagnostic process work better and improve the chances for an accurate diagnosis, we will examine how medical diagnostics works in general and, more specifically, how it is applied in the realm of stealth infections.

3. How Medical Conditions and Stealth Germs Are Diagnosed

How Diagnoses Are Made . . . or Missed

As you read this book you may ask yourself the question: Could you really have an undiagnosed chronic infection in your body when you have had regular checkups, laboratory tests, and possibly even a total body scan, and your doctor told you that "nothing" (meaning "nothing abnormal") was found? The answer is yes.

The Problem

To understand how such a contradiction is possible, we need to remind ourselves that certain chronic, low-grade infections may not cause symptoms that most of us would associate with infection. For example, stomach ulcers and cancer of the cervix, both of which have recently been conclusively attributed to chronic infections, do not cause traditional symptoms of infection. As a result, neither the patient nor the doctor would start the evaluation of such problems by considering or looking for an infection.

Let us understand how medical diagnoses are made to see how this can be remedied.

If medical diagnosis were straightforward and simple, computers would be doing it routinely. However, over the last couple of decades it has become clear that attempts to use computers to make medical diagnoses have largely failed for reasons that are detailed in the next section. If computers are unable to do it well, then it is not surprising that patients and doctors might also fail to correctly diagnose existing medical conditions.

The advent of total body scans, which promised to find every abnormal bodily condition, generated hope for identifying undiagnosed and hidden illnesses. This hope was soon dashed as total body scans failed to diagnose many medical conditions. Still, many continue to hold the erroneous belief that if they can just get the right tests, they will get a foolproof diagnosis. Sadly, tests don't make diagnoses. Tests often provide very important clues and sometimes proof, but ultimately it is the diagnostician who must make the diagnosis after he or she has examined all the information, and suddenly "gets the picture."

How easy is it to miss a diagnosis where an infectious organism is lurking? Consider the following case study: An older patient is brought to an urgent care center by his pregnant daughter because of rather severe pain on the left side of the chest. He is in excellent health, and a year earlier had a checkup, laboratory tests, a cardiac stress test, and a total body scan. At the urgent care center, an electrocardiogram (EKG) is taken, and the computer indicates there are abnormalities. The doctor confirms the questionable findings. An X-ray of the chest, ribs, and spine is taken. The X-ray reveals a partial compression fracture of a vertebra near the nerve root that corresponds to the region of the pain. There are two possible leading diagnoses: The first is heart attack, in which case hospitalization is required. The second possibility is that the pain is caused by the partly collapsed vertebra, which may need to be "fixed."

A Lurking Stealth Infection Erupts

This cautious diagnostician, however, questions the patient further and finds that his symptoms came on gradually, not suddenly, and that they do not relate to movement or position or activity. The patient also indicates that the skin is unusually sensitive along the area where the pain is felt. Tapping over the ribs and the area of the spine that appears abnormal on the X-ray does not produce pain. The patient does not have the washed-out feeling often reported during a heart attack. The initial blood test, which looks for chemical evidence of a heart attack, is negative, and other blood and urine tests also come back normal. However, the skin over the chest is indeed very sensitive to light touch. The diagnostician correctly suspects and concludes that the patient is about to develop a painful skin eruption caused by the stealth germ *Varicella zoster*, called shingles. This virus has been present, but dormant, in this patient's body for decades. It went into hiding after causing chicken pox during his childhood.

The doctor looks at the patient's previous X-rays and EKGs, and finds that the partially crushed vertebra was present on an X-ray two years earlier, and was caused by an old injury. The patient's EKG changes are the same as those noted in prior years, and are considered a normal variant. The patient is carefully observed, and a few days later he indeed erupts with the classic shingles rash and blisters along the tender skin line. To erase any doubts, though this is not usually necessary, a test of the blister fluid confirmed the presence of the *Varicella zoster* virus. The initial EKG and X-ray tests not only did not prove the diagnosis, but were misleading rather than helpful. An inexperienced diagnostician might have admitted the patient to the hospital for treatment of the wrong problem at considerable cost to the patient. Furthermore, the pregnant daughter would have been unwittingly exposed to the virus. Though the tests did not show it, and the patient and family did not suspect it, the doctor made the correct diagnosis. He saved the patient the unnecessary expense of hospitalization, and protected the daughter from exposure to chicken pox.

The doctor clearly suspected and correctly diagnosed shingles even before the final clue (the rash) arrived, and placed other misleading clues into perspective. Was there a test that proved it? Only after the fact. By knowing the condition well, even in the absence of tests, this physician correctly diagnosed and successfully treated this potentially mysterious but well-known infectious medical condition. Is this realistic? Should a patient take the doctor's word for such a diagnosis in the absence of some conclusive test result?

If blood analyzers, computers, and million-dollar scanners cannot diagnose medical problems, how does the diagnostician arrive at the correct answer? And how could this perfectly healthy individual carry a disease-causing virus without feeling it, then suddenly without warning be attacked and made ill by the same virus that has been traveling with him for decades without causing any disturbance whatsoever? Could there be other such germs in his body lurking and lying in wait for the right opportunity to cause disease? Evidently so.

A Piece of the Diagnostic Puzzle

One way to understand medical diagnostics is to compare it to solving jigsaw puzzles (other analogies may be a game of "name that tune" or attempting to identify a movie by hearing or seeing parts of it). Each disease is like a jigsaw puzzle: The picture of the disease is made up of dozens of puzzle pieces, consisting of symptoms, signs, laboratory test results, and other findings. The process of diagnosis consists of gathering as many bits of information as possible about a patient's medical condition, then assembling the puzzle pieces systematically into a still or moving picture that makes medical sense. The diagnostician assembles information by taking a medical history followed by physical examination, followed by laboratory and other tests. The assembled information is then compared to all known medical conditions and diseases. The comparison is done rapidly but systematically by a series of "what if?" or "could it be?" questions. This process is called hypothesis testing. Finally the best match is selected, and a name is assigned to the picture that emerges.

As in solving a jigsaw puzzle, the first step is to identify prominent or key bits of information (think of them as the corner and frame pieces of the puzzle) so that the diagnostician can begin to understand the outlines of the picture that emerges. Critical to this is to really understand in clear and simple terms what is the main symptom that is bothering or concerning the patient, and certain judgments are made about what the critical information may be. When the framework is in place, other pieces begin to fit more readily. When some pieces don't fit, the good diagnostician sets them aside, and goes back to look for missing pieces. He or she may ask specifically for a suspected missing piece of information. After a while, all of a sudden there is the moment when the diagnostician gets the whole picture. Such is the process whereby most medical diagnoses are made. This is why medical diagnostics is referred to as an art, though medicine itself is science.

Just as there are some people who are very good at doing jigsaw puzzles, there are also exceptionally good diagnosticians. Surprisingly, human beings are better at doing jigsaw puzzles (as well as medical diagnostics) than computers. What an experienced human being can do is assign relative importance to various bits of information based on experience, hunches, sight, smell, and intuition. A good diagnostician is distinguished not by how quick or how smart he is, but how experienced, how careful, and how methodical he or she is in sorting pieces of information, and how well he or she knows all of the several thousand medical jigsaw puzzle pictures we call diseases which allows him or her to judge the relevance of certain bits of information. The really perceptive diagnostician even keeps alert to the likelihood that he or she may be encountering some previously unknown or unnamed disease, perhaps due to some infectious organism that has not yet been identified.

However . . . It's Not Quite That Easy

All of this would still be relatively simple if the diagnostician were asked to work on a single puzzle with a limited number of pieces. Such is often the case in young patients, where one single medical condition will account for all the patient's symptoms. This is less likely to apply to most middle-aged adults and especially older persons. In such patients, diagnosis becomes vastly more complicated. There are often numerous medical conditions present side-by-side, each of which can correspond to a complete medical jigsaw puzzle picture. A single piece or symptom, such as headache, may be part of the solution to several of the puzzles and part of several constellations of symptoms, and pieces of various puzzles may get jumbled with others. Now the diagnostician must do something akin to solving a stack of jigsaw puzzles simultaneously, where each piece will eventually need to be correctly sorted into one of the several pictures.

Making things even more complicated is the fact that most medical conditions are not static. They evolve over time, and may look different at different stages. In this way, medical diagnosis may also be likened to catching bits and pieces of a movie and being asked to guess the title of the particular movie that is playing.

Complicating the process further is the genetic makeup of each patient. Not all persons are perfectly normal, if there is such a thing. Well-known diseases may manifest themselves in a distorted fashion in a person with inborn abnormalities or in someone with a coexisting medical condition. For example, a broken bone may cause no pain in a person who has a loss of sensation in part of the body due to prior stroke or nerve injury.

Medications can cloud the diagnostic picture still further. For example, persons who are taking prednisone, a synthetic corticosteroid preparation, may not have a fever despite the presence of an infection that usually causes fever. Someone already on strong pain medicines may not feel the pain of an appendix attack. The jigsaw puzzle picture for an identical medical problem may be rather different for various individuals. Yet the diagnostician must see beyond this, and still correctly get the picture.

Simple puzzles are easy to solve without much training. Most parents and grandparents can reliably recognize an insect bite, pinkeye, or even gout in the manner of "name that tune" after hearing just a few notes of a song. However, a low-grade, smoldering problem hidden behind a dozen or more coexisting conditions will not be apparent to the layperson or even to some professionals. This situation calls for methodical and thoughtful analysis of information. The diagnostician has to keep looking at the pieces of information over and over again, reassembling them and re-sorting them, raising and examining various hypotheses, in order to find the key pieces that may distinguish one picture from the other.

Laboratory Tests

In addition to obtaining a complete medical history and an examination of the patient, quite often routine laboratory tests are done as part of the problem-solving process. When a "complete blood count" or a "comprehensive chemistry panel" are ordered, most patients assume that these tests indeed provide complete and comprehensive information. However, the names of these tests are misleading. In truth, there is no such thing as a comprehensive laboratory test that tests for everything. Routine laboratory tests are basic screening methods, which accomplish a limited search for certain common conditions such as diabetes, kidney disease, liver disease, anemia, and so on. When routine tests fail to deliver conclusive answers, the diagnostician will order specific additional laboratory tests in order to obtain specific clues about particular conditions, especially suspected hidden infections. Which additional tests the physician chooses to obtain, however, is influenced by preconceived notions about the problem at hand. Determining which tests will lead to the most reliable answer in the minimum necessary steps and at minimum expense is also part of the art of medicine, and distinguishes a superb diagnostician from an average one.

Where Mistakes Are Made

Unfortunately, when pressed for time, some diagnosticians may try to play "name that tune" just as a layperson would, and leap to conclusions based on the first few bits of information they receive. Others jump to a diagnosis after seeing only part of the puzzle, and neglect to ask for added information or consider other possible solutions. Other diagnosticians make the mistake of assembling some pieces of the puzzle initially, but then failing to take them apart and reassemble them later when they find pieces that don't seem to fit. Instead of starting over, they try to force the rest of the puzzle to fit.

Another common mistake in the diagnostic process is that physicians often quickly interrupt the patient when the patient is first describing his or her complaint. Such interruptions usually are inspired by an attempt to clarify things, but often such interruption distracts the patient, who then is kept from explaining details that would have been critical to obtaining the complete picture needed for the correct diagnosis.

The Patient's Role in Diagnosis and Misdiagnosis

The diagnostic process, of course, involves not only the diagnostician, but also the patient. Some people are embarrassed to bring up certain issues, and therefore in giving their medical history leave out vital information that may contain important clues. Others instinctively suspect that it is important to present all of the information, no matter how trivial it may seem, and that leaving out even one single piece with potential significance can lead to a missed diagnosis. For this reason, these patients provide an excessively detailed accounting of everything they have experienced over a period of months, resulting in an overwhelming amount jumbled and unedited information. Other patients may try to help the doctor by presenting their own diagnostic impressions and conclusions about what they suspect is causing their symptoms ("I have arthritis of the hip") rather than presenting the symptoms themselves ("the side of my thigh hurts when I walk"). This may steer the doctor to a wrong diagnosis. Providing organized, unbiased, factual information and observations is usually the best way to help the diagnostician to arrive at the right answer.

Of course, the dilemma is the same for both patient and doctor: Unless you know what you are looking for, it is difficult to know what information is relevant and what isn't. One needs to know what diagnoses even come into consideration before one will know the relevance of various items. Often we don't even know what the right question to ask is until we get close to the answer. Indeed, this uncertainty is the reason why the sorting process needs to be methodical and why experienced diagnosticians are usually better than novices.

The Unknown

Another challenging aspect of making correct diagnoses is that there are still some unidentified conditions, infections, and diseases. There are also some known but rare and exotic conditions, which the diagnostician may be only marginally aware of. Some of the diseases associated with stealth infections were only recently understood. When a disease is not yet known or described in medical books or journals, even the best diagnostician will miss the proper diagnosis and treatment.

These complexities are the reasons why some persons may have an ongoing medical condition that was not properly diagnosed, despite the fact that they have regularly sought medical care. Most of their obvious problems were likely identified correctly. However, some not-so-obvious underlying conditions may still be scattered as pieces, yet to be assembled into another whole picture. Fortunately, there are ways to collaborate with one's physician so that if there is some undiagnosed infectious condition in the body, the likelihood of finding and treating it will be improved. The patient shouldn't expect a computer to give the diagnosis. Old-fashioned detective work will still have to provide the answers.

If you suspect that there is an infectious organism in your system, or that you have some other undiagnosed condition that might account for some problems you have been experiencing, sit down with your doctor, or ask for a consultation with a specialist. Ask them to start from the beginning, without any preconceived notions, to take a fresh look at the evidence.

But isn't there a simpler and more efficient way of doing this? Wouldn't a total body scan provide the answer?

How About a Total Body Scan?

In this high-tech age, there must be a better way to make a diagnosis than attempting to solve a jigsaw puzzle. High-tech scans have arrived, such as CT (computerized tomography) and MRI (magnetic resonance imaging) scans. Surely these technologies can be relied on to detect any problem, including lurking infections in the body?

Total Body Scans Miss Many Diagnoses

Unfortunately, they cannot. There is no single test that will find all abnormal conditions in the human body. In fact, conventional total body scans are generally of little help in uncovering chronic low-grade smoldering infections.

Nonetheless, high-tech full-body scans (usually done with CT scanners) are widely promoted to those desiring more than the usual information about their health. However, for the reasons given below, these scans are not recommended for health screening by public health organizations such as the American Cancer Society, the American College of Radiology and the U.S. Food and Drug Administration, and are usually not covered by health insurance or Medicare for general health screening purposes. Still, patients often ask physicians whether they should pay out-of-pocket for one of these scans.

Are full-body scans useful? The answer is not a simple yes or no. The issue is not whether such scans are able to detect hidden conditions, but rather which ones, and how reliable their findings are. Basically healthy patients without any symptoms or complaints often wish to undergo a scan to reassure themselves that they are indeed completely healthy. But even if the scan shows everything to be normal, it's not necessarily so. Infections that may be about to erupt, such as shingles, are not detectable with such a tool. While certain scans are rather good at identifying coronary artery disease, one can walk away from a totally normal body scan or heart scan and suddenly drop dead of a cardiac arrhythmia, which the scan will not predict. A normal scan can also miss a leaky heart valve, which may require taking preventive antibiotics with every dental cleaning. One could also have a normal scan yet have extremely high blood pressure, diabetes, AIDS, or leukemia. Likewise, such scans almost never detect chronic infections such as syphilis, hepatitis, stomach ulcer bacteria, early cancer of the cervix, or a low-grade bladder infection to name a few.

Some persons with certain undiagnosed symptoms hope that a scan will give them a conclusive answer to the cause of their problem. They may be disappointed. For example, a person experiencing severe pain in the neck and shoulders may be told that her scan shows a bone spur or a partially slipped disk. Even though the scan indeed shows such findings, the real cause of the pain may not be the spur or the disk, but polymyalgia rheumatica (PMR), an inflammatory muscle condition. All the scans will miss this potentially serious and dangerous condition, which can only be detected using a particular blood test, called the erythrocyte sedimentation rate test (see Glossary). This test is not usually included in routine blood testing, and must be specifically ordered by your doctor if the condition is suspected.

Even though scans miss many important conditions, proponents suggest they are valuable for finding otherwise unsuspected cancer. Unfortunately, there are problems here as well. Scans cannot detect early cancer of the cervix, only a Pap smear does. Skin cancer, including melanoma, won't be discovered by the scan, only by inspection of the skin. Cancer of the blood, such as leukemia, won't be identified either. Even small cancerous growths in the colon may not reliably be found by a scan, only through a sigmoidoscopic or colonoscopic examination.

Furthermore, a normal scan today doesn't guarantee that a person won't have a newly formed cancer of the pancreas by the next year.

What if a scan does show something? X-rays, including CT scans, are "shadow pictures" and do not prove whether a spot is cancerous or non-cancerous, infectious or noninfectious. A small spot found on the lung may be scar tissue from an earlier chest infection, and of little or no consequence. Alternately, it could be cancer in the early stage, or a lymph node harboring tuberculosis. The X-ray cannot conclusively tell what it is. There may not be any way to prove the diagnosis except to biopsy or remove the questionable part of the lung. Many physicians and public health agencies are concerned that large numbers of scans indeed show such scars from old events or injuries, or show various other harmless cysts or malformations. As a result, substantial numbers of patients may be taken to surgery or for invasive biopsy only to be told that the finding noted on X-ray was of no health consequence.

Even if one decides that it is beneficial to have such a scan, it is unclear how often the scans should be repeated, at what age they should begin, and at what age they are no longer useful.

No Substitute for Detective Work

If a total body scan cannot give a comprehensive answer about your health, then what can? As we discussed earlier, the most reliable medical diagnosis is made by a trained diagnostician using a combination of information obtained from the history of your condition, a physical examination, followed by laboratory tests, scans, and other examinations. No single part of this sequence of steps is foolproof, or can stand alone. It is the synthesis of all the information that leads to a final, reliable answer.

Body scans do not substitute for thoughtful detective work. They are only one item in the toolbox of the master diagnostician. If responsible professional agencies are to approve the use of such scans for routine screening purposes, the tests must be shown to provide not only interesting, but also reliably useful information that will benefit the person's health. Proof of efficacy must be obtained through outcome studies, which are the cornerstone of evidence-based medicine.

There is nothing particularly wrong with these scans, though some expose the patient to a significant dose of radiation. Some patients may also have adverse reactions to the contrast agents infused into the blood in order to improve and highlight the X-ray or MRI image. Scans give limited answers to limited questions. What role, if any, they should play in periodic checkups remains to be determined. Proponents point out that sometimes such scans uncover something truly important: a diagnosis that has not been suspected. On occasion this is true. However, it is not clear if this happened in the case of patients who had a recent thorough checkup with a good diagnostician, or patients who went in for the test without having seen a doctor for years.

A total body scan could be done to rule out certain other possible problems, but usually won't help you discover a hidden infection. When seeking answers to suspected medical problems, one should not rely on a single test, but seek a thorough and detailed evaluation.

What, then, is involved in obtaining a thorough and detailed evaluation?

Collaborating with Your Doctor to Get a Diagnosis

The importance of arriving at the correct diagnosis should be clear by now. Once the accurate and detailed diagnosis is made, it is quite straightforward to look up the recommended treatment in a reference book, journal, or on the Internet. In what way can you, as a patient, or your doctor, optimally contribute to the success of the diagnostic process?

Medical conditions are considered to be "diagnosed" when given a medical name or label by the doctor. However, even when a name such as irritable bowel syndrome, dermatitis, gastritis, or asthmatic bronchitis has been assigned, an infectious stealth germ that could be the underlying cause may still have been overlooked. Therefore, even if your condition has been properly labeled, it may not have been completely diagnosed. Certain diagnoses may need to be taken to a higher level. For example, if you have an ulcer, is it due to stress, ingested substances, or a particular infectious organism? If you have irritable bowel syndrome, could it be due to lactose intolerance or an infectious organism? If you have dermatitis, is it compounded by an infectious organism or due to an underlying infection? Just because some condition is assigned a diagnostic label, it does not necessarily mean that the true underlying process or triggering cause of the condition has been identified or understood. In such cases, treatment may merely manage the symptoms and neglect to target the underlying cause.

It will take a collaborative effort between you and your physician to get the most accurate and complete diagnosis. The method outlined below is relevant not only to infectious conditions, but can be applied to solving any other ongoing or long-standing medical problem.

If you have a simple, straightforward problem, it is easy to present the details to your doctor and get a quick answer. However, if you have more complex, persistent problems, it is important that you are organized and well prepared. You will need to proceed through the sequence of steps most doctors take: (1) history, (2) physical examination, (3) laboratory and other tests, (4) diagnosis, and finally (5) treatment.

Making Your Case

You, the patient, are a vital part of the diagnostic process. This does not mean that you are expected to make the diagnosis. Don't try to be your own diagnostician. Don't be too quick to jump to conclusions about cause and effect. Don't expect information on the Internet to give your diagnosis; looking up information is vastly different from making diagnoses. A single laboratory test won't do it, either, except in some simple cases. If you have a reasonable suspicion of what you may have, you can help the diagnostic process move in the right direction. It is fair, and in fact useful, to raise a question at the right time with your doctor about a particular diagnosis that you may suspect. But don't try to jump to conclusions too early in the process.

If you are uncertain about the cause of your symptoms, your job is to present your case to the diagnostician and present it right. The doctor's job is to "get the picture" and get it right.

If you have a complicated problem, you might be wondering where you can find a master diagnostician. Unfortunately, such a specialty is not listed in the directory of physicians. Even if you don't know such a master diagnostician, most careful doctors can rise to the occasion if you help them.

The first thing you can do to help the doctor is to describe and outline your complaint. Think of a simple and concise statement that tells what is bothering you. This may not be as simple as it sounds. The symptoms of chronic ailments may be vague. Nevertheless, you will need to describe as accurately as you can the way you feel now that is different from the way you felt when well.

It is equally important that you detail how your symptoms have evolved over time. Whether your doctor will consider or suspect a particular diagnosis depends on how you present the information in your initial interview. It is important that the right diagnosis be considered from the very beginning.

You should prepare. Just like an attorney in court, you have to present your case properly in order to be heard; otherwise your case may be dismissed without a hearing. And if you hope that the culprit of the diagnostic mystery will be recognized in one hearing, you have to tell the story systematically. There is a method to accomplishing this.

Keep your presentation brief and to the point. Keep it focused, with a concise timeline, and present all necessary information. A brief, well-written summary outline is an excellent way to accomplish this. When talking, you must not overwhelm your doctor by providing too many pieces too fast, or by providing information in a scattered way. The doctor's understanding of your history must come first. It is often the key to deciding what tests are likely to be useful in proving or disproving certain diagnoses. Even though you think a particular test may be helpful, do not start with "Shouldn't I get an MRI?" Begin by outlining and describing your symptoms. Tests are the last step toward arriving at a diagnosis and need to be specifically chosen to uncover or rule out suspected conditions.

In preparing for your visit, you should gather your previous medical records, including your blood tests, scans, X-rays, and chart notes from other doctors or specialists. However, unless specifically requested, do not give these to your diagnostician at the start of the consultation, but toward the end. Doing it in this way will prevent biasing or possibly misleading the examining doctor with the opinions of other physicians, and will enable your current doctor to look at you with a fresh eye.

Do not start with leading questions (such as "Doctor, don't you really think I have tuberculosis?"). Do not bias the examiner at the beginning with your own conclusions about what you think may be ailing you. Wait toward the end of the interview to present your suspicions. After a tentative diagnostic impression is rendered by your physician, you should have opportunity to raise and discuss other possibilities, and in fact this may be quite useful.

Perhaps it has been your experience that such a process doesn't work because the doctor is in too much of a hurry? Unfortunately, that may happen more often than we would like. If you know that you have a complicated problem, one way to anticipate this is to request an extended re-examination or an extended consultation, rather than a simple office visit when you arrange your appointment. The physician will then be more open to a slower and more detailed problem-solving session.

Here are some general guidelines on how to interact with your doctor. To begin with, let us try to understand how the process and doctors work.

A Visit to Your Doctor

A visit to the doctor is often a frustrating experience. Surveys have shown that during the usual office visit, doctors generally interrupt the patient within the first half minute. One survey showed interruptions within eighteen seconds!

To minimize the chance of being cut off, you should prepare a brief written summary of your symptoms and problems, although there is always a small chance that the doctor may not look at it. Be aware that most doctors in medical school learned about a condition called by the French name *le maladie du petit papier*—"the malady of the small piece of paper." In years past it was generally believed by physicians that persons who wrote out a long list of symptoms on a small piece of paper were likely suffering from psychosomatic or neurotic conditions. However, if you bring a concise, focused medical summary, your doctor will likely use it. Make the doctor aware that you are simply trying to present complete and organized information. You can also point out that your well-written history may save time and cost, since he or she won't need to have it transcribed for the record.

How Doctors Process Information

Most doctors use the time-honored "chief complaint, history, physical examination, laboratory tests, then diagnosis" sequence in problem-solving. Therefore, expect your story to be considered in the same order, but keep it concise. Consider using the sample form provided in the Appendix to organize the information. Presenting your story will usually generate questions by the doctor, and some discussion and clarification of the information. Ideally this will be followed by a physical examination with special focus on the area of your body that is raising concern. Finally, laboratory tests may be ordered. The tests are usually selected specifically to rule in or rule out the probable cause of your problems, and to establish a working diagnosis.

The medical narrative you prepare should include:
1. Main symptom(s) (chief complaint)
2. Timeline (history of present illness)
3. Prior problems and operations (past medical and surgical history)
4a. Medicines and substances you take or use (medicines and habits)
4b. Allergies or adverse reactions
5. Medical problems that run in your family (family history)
6. Miscellaneous other symptoms (review of systems)
7. Your suspicion about what may be ailing you (possible diagnosis)

Main Symptom(s) (Chief Complaint)

"The main symptom I have that bothers/concerns me is" . . . Use your own words to describe the most notable way in which you don't feel right, or the symptoms that bother you, such as headache, fevers, sweats, fatigue, neck pain, belly pains, palpitations, itchy rash, diarrhea, swollen joints, chronic cough, or not feeling well in general. Start with the most prominent symptoms, and make a short list in order of their importance.

When indicating your chief complaint do not try to give a diagnosis, such as "I think I have chronic tuberculosis." Say "I have chronic cough or fever or blood in my saliva." Your suspicion about a specific condition should be raised after the diagnostician has had an initial chance to consider the significance of your symptoms and findings on his or her own.

What is a symptom? How do we know when something doesn't feel right or act right? Most of us know when we feel normal. Describe how you are feeling different than when you last felt well. Symptoms are not visible. Only you can tell how you feel and what you feel, but this is very important for the diagnostician to understand! Signs are those findings that can be seen or heard by the patient or the observer, such as lumps, bumps, swelling, redness, rashes, and so on. Make note of these as well.

Timeline (History of Present Illness)

Give a description or outline of what has happened. Start at the beginning when you first started to not feel right, even if you are not entirely sure whether it has anything to do with your current ailment. Indicate what has happened, but do not try to conclude why. Your assessment of cause and effect may be misleading or inaccurate. Describe each complaint separately.

Since some conditions evolve like the plot of a movie, you need to lay out your story in a similar way, but keep it brief and focused. "I last felt well . . . It all started when . . . The first thing I noticed was . . . The next thing that happened was . . . After I was treated with . . . I was better/not better after taking the medicine . . . Most recently it got even worse . . . I had further tests and treatments . . . Now I am experiencing . . ."

Remember, it's easier for someone to recognize a movie when they see it in sequence rather than seeing bits of it jumbled together. Don't start with the ending, even if you believe that the ending says it all. There is no need to give precise dates, but rather a rough timeline.

Prior Problems and Operations (Past Medical and Surgical History)

Make a brief numbered list of conditions that are likely not directly related to your current concerns but which were previously identified or diagnosed:

1. Medical conditions (pneumonia, kidney stone, malaria) with approximate dates.
2. Surgeries or procedures (appendix removed, hysterectomy, blood transfusion, breast biopsy, pinning of broken bone) with dates.
3. Significant accidents and injuries (such as concussion or ruptured spleen) with approximate dates.
4a. Medicines and Substances You Take or Use (Medicines and Habits) Include a complete list of
    (i) prescription medications
    (ii) nonprescription medications
    (iii) vitamins, minerals, and supplements
    (iv) herbal preparations
    (v) recreational substances, including alcohol or tobacco
    (vi) prior exposure to toxic substances or radiation
4b. Allergies or Adverse Reactions
    Include nature of untoward reactions or true allergies to
    (i) medicines
    (ii) chemicals
    (iii) foods
    (iv) plants or materials (poison oak, adhesive tape, latex)
    (v) insect bites

Note: Not all reactions to substances are allergies. Nausea and vomiting when taking codeine or erythromycin are adverse side effects, not allergies.

Medical Problems That Run in Your Family (Family History)

List significant medical problems of blood relatives including parents, siblings, grandparents, children, aunts, uncles, cousins, etc. You should also include significant contagious diseases of close friends and associates who are not blood relatives.

Miscellaneous Other Symptoms (Review of Systems)

List any other minor findings which you think have doubtful relevance to your current complaint, such as fungus on your toenails, a bunion, dental problems, and so on. Begin the list with the top of your head and continue until you reach your toes. Some of these complaints might be relevant to the problem at hand without you being aware of it.

Your Suspicion About What May Be Ailing You (Possible Diagnosis)

If you have a particular idea or worry about what your diagnosis may be, this is a good place to state your thoughts about what may be ailing you. "I am concerned/I believe I may have . . ." It is useful to add this at the end.

Often a patient is seen for a problem, such as bad headaches. The doctor makes the correct diagnosis and explains it, but the patient does not appear relieved. It is revealing to both when the doctor asks, "Did you have a particular concern about what your symptoms may mean?" The patient says, "Yes. Could I have a brain tumor? A friend of mine just died of a brain tumor, and had similar symptoms." You will receive a more direct and relevant answer about your symptoms if such a concern is made clear. Stating your specific concern will also help refocus the discussion to the problem at hand.

To Complete the Process (Working Diagnosis)

This is the time when the doctor should examine you, then formulate and tell you his or her initial impression and opinion of the probable cause of your problems, called the "working diagnosis" in medical terms.

If the doctor doesn't volunteer such an impression, then ask: "What do you think is causing my problem and how do we plan to prove it or treat it? And could it be due to . . . ?"

Now, the doctor may suggest laboratory tests, X-rays, or scans in order to obtain further information. If such tests are done, you should ask to receive the results, or else schedule a follow-up visit to go over the findings and make plans for treatment and management. At the follow-up visit, again consider using the worksheet in the Appendix if you still have a question about your diagnosis and treatment plans.

This is how to approach collaborating with most doctors. Occasionally, despite everyone's best intentions, the process will not work. Don't be discouraged. Go by the old maxim: If at first you don't succeed, try and try again, perhaps with another diagnostician or a specialist. If you think you have a significant problem, do not give up too soon.

With this understanding of the issues of infection, and the diagnostic process and how to make it work, it is time once again to ask the basic question about stealth infections: Could they be the hidden source of your present or future chronic ailment?

Smoldering Stealth Infections in Your Body

It is time to pose the question about the relationship between stealth germs and your symptoms. Do you in fact carry a stealth germ? If you do, is it causing none, or only certain of your symptoms?

If a germ that normally doesn't belong in healthy human beings winds up in your system without creating a noticeable disturbance, is that necessarily something you should worry about? The body is host to billions and billions of germs. Could you develop a newly found symbiotic relationship with one more, so the organism doesn't bother you, just as the body accommodates its own natural flora?

This appears to happen in some cases. Individuals who carry abnormal germs without exhibiting illness are called asymptomatic carriers. Carrying the chicken pox—shingles (*Varicella-zoster*) virus is an obvious example. It is often assumed that asymptomatic carriers have reached a symbiotic relationship with the "carried" organism. But is that really the case?

Some travelers upon returning from travel adventures abroad are found to carry *Blastocystis hominis* or *Entamoeba coli* in their bowels. They have hardly any symptoms except for being somewhat more gassy than usual. They may be told that these organisms are nonpathogenic germs and require no treatment. They are told that many people in the tropics chronically carry these organisms without any sign of trouble. But will carrying such a germ in one's bowels for the next few decades truly be harmless and nonpathogenic? Could these organisms ultimately cause low-grade damage to the bowels or some sudden trouble when this former traveler takes corticosteroids or requires cancer chemotherapy?

Accumulating Evidence of Harm from Stealth Germs
There is growing evidence that colonization by germs that do not normally belong in the system generally does *not* result in a symbiotic relationship with the host, and in fact may account for large numbers of conditions and diseases previously not attributed to infections. There is an emerging consensus suggesting that in the relationship between stealth infections and chronic disease it is just as much of a mistake to underestimate a causal connection as it is to overestimate one. Stealth germ organisms are probably best avoided. If you wind up harboring one of these stealth germs, it is best to try to be cured of it.

The Problems of Cause and Effect
Physicians are traditionally cautious and reluctant to conclude a cause-and-effect association between an organism that is found in a certain location in the body, and symptoms that may develop some time later in that location or somewhere else. They rightfully adhere to the well-known maxim that "correlation does not mean causation." As a result, they have traditionally underestimated such connections.

A scientifically proven cause-and-effect relationship between germ and disease is difficult to establish. Even when there are clear-cut signs of infection, the newly found presence of a particular germ at that location does not establish beyond question a true cause-and-effect relationship. Even outside of the realm of medicine there is the well-known logical fallacy of causality, "ergo hoc, ergo propter hoc." Just because event B follows event A, it does not necessarily mean that A caused B to occur.

Influenza, which is caused by the influenza virus, is a well-known historical example of the mistaken attribution of an illness to a particular germ. After viral influenza infection sets in, many persons' lungs soon become overrun also by the bacterial organism *Haemophilus influenzae*, so named by Dr. Richard Pfeiffer, who first identified it over a hundred years ago. Because viruses were difficult to detect in those days, finding this bacterial organism in the lungs of many influenza victims mistakenly led to the notion that *H. influenzae* was the actual cause of influenza, rather than an opportunistic organism that overran the lung surface after it was injured by the virus. It took some time for this misconception to be corrected.

It was known for many decades that both the surface of stomach ulcers and the stomach lining of many persons without ulcers were colonized by *Helicobacter pylori*. It is also known that sores or wounds on the skin are colonized by various organisms. That leads to the following questions: Which comes first? Does a stomach ulcer form, then certain germs colonize the abnormal surface? Or do the germs somehow cause the sore to form? Similarly, does a skin sore form and then become colonized by organisms such as *Pseudomonas aeruginosa*, or does a "pseudomonas infection" cause the sore to develop? If someone develops impetigo, does he or she acquire a colony of a certain strain of staphylococcus bacteria that causes the crusty boils of impetigo to form? Or is there something wrong with that person's skin or immunity that allows these germs to proliferate? If you eradicate such germs, will the sore heal more readily? How do you prove cause and effect?

Scientifically minded physicians require strong evidence to be convinced of cause-and-effect relationships between a symptom or symptoms and a particular infection. For example, those who carry the herpes simplex virus tend to have occasional outbreaks of a cold sore near the mouth or genitals. Is the presence of the virus also why some of these persons never feel well, or why they have headaches or stomachaches or other skin rashes or frequent bladder infections? Or do most people with herpesvirus generally feel fine, except for the few days when the cold sore appears? Most of the time, those infected with herpesvirus are believed to have no symptoms other than the episodic skin sores from the herpesvirus. However, there is evidence that carrying certain other of the herpesviruses (there are eight major different types of human herpesviruses) may be the cause of such unlikely consequences as sudden-onset Bell's palsy or sudden "unexplained" hearing loss. Yet very few who carry the virus develop these consequences.

When we consider such erratic results from an infection, we should remember that no two persons are genetically and immunologically identical and therefore each may have a different reaction to the germs they carry (even identical twins may have different exposures over time). Also, they may not carry the same number ("load") of organisms. We must avoid generalization. Some may have no symptoms, some minimal symptoms, and some significant symptoms. As indicated before, individual variations of responses to illness are one of the complexities of medical diagnosis.

In the case of long-term smoldering infection, and in the absence of the classic signs and symptoms (fever, chills, malaise, discharge, swelling) it is unlikely that patient or doctor would think of attributing nonspecific symptoms to colonization or infestation by some germ within the body. Even though physicians learn in medical school about chronic syphilis infection being the "great masquerader" that can cause all sorts of symptoms not suggestive of a chronic infection, until recently most physicians did not apply the same degree of suspicion to other infectious organisms. Yet the only signs of stealth germ infection may be subtle: the person may not feel quite right, without being truly ill, or have episodic "odd" events such as episodic belly pains, a sensitive stomach, or even sudden hearing loss.

The Needed Proof

When the germ theory of disease was first accepted, rules were laid down that stated specific premises that must be satisfied to scientifically prove that an organism causes a particular disease or condition. These rules were first described by the German microbiologist Robert Koch, who discovered the bacterial organism that causes tuberculosis (*Mycobacterium tuberculosis*: "Koch's bacillus"). These rules are known as "Koch's Postulates" and are still used today:

The germ must be present in every case of the disease.

The germ must be isolated from the host and grown in a laboratory dish.

The disease must be reproduced when a pure culture of the germ is inoculated into a healthy susceptible host.

The same germ must be recovered again from the experimentally infected host.

These rules are very useful to laboratory scientists and biologists studying acute infections. However, there are obvious practical problems in following these rules in day-to-day medical practices, especially when dealing with long-term smoldering infections. Even Dr. Koch knew that certain germs that grow in human cells do not grow easily in a laboratory dish, and therefore are very difficult to test. Furthermore, while such experiments can be done in laboratory animals, they cannot be done on patients because deliberately infecting or re-infecting a person just to prove a diagnosis almost never passes muster in a risk-benefit evaluation and, more importantly, raises serious ethical considerations.

Yet for doctors with a scientific bent, such proof is mandatory for definitive acceptance of the cause-and effect relationship between a specific infection and disease. The lack of such proof is the reason why many doctors have been reluctant to attribute various ailments to particular stealth infections. However the trend is now shifting toward a less rigid, but more practical criteria of considering the overwhelming preponderance of the evidence. Of course, cautious medical scientists point out, that just as in legal proceedings, overwhelming evidence can sometimes be wrong. True. But waiting for absolute proof can also lead to the dismissal of charges against a truly guilty party, which can be an equally great mistake.

Part of the reason the Nobel Prize was awarded to the Australian physicians Barry J. Marshall, M.D., and J. Robin Warren, M.D., for proving that *Helicobacter pylori* caused stomach ulcers, was because they (very nearly) satisfied the requirements of Koch's postulates by running the experiment with Dr. Marshall as the host who deliberately ingested a colony of *H. pylori* organisms. At his own risk they proved the cause-and-effect relationship between this particular germ and stomach ulcers. Thankfully, *H. pylori* is treatable with antibiotics, and not life-threatening or untreatable like the SARS or Ebola viruses. Nevertheless, because of ethical barriers to long-term human experiments with this curable bacterium, the strongly suspected link between stomach cancer and long-standing untreated *H. pylori* infection has not, and likely will not, be proven in a similar direct experiment.

Even beyond proving this one disease-germ association, the huge significance of the work of Drs. Marshall and Warren was the remarkable demonstration of the idea that a stealth germ can cause a medical condition without giving obvious signs of infection. The work of these doctors heightened our awareness of the concept of the existence of stealth germs, and opened the door to further study of the role of other germs in diseases not formerly considered to be caused by infections. *H. pylori* put us on notice that even if a person feels well and has few symptoms suggestive of an infection, there may be pathogenic germs slowly smoldering in certain tissues, waiting to do harm in the future. Some of these germs may take a decade or even much longer before they reveal the final damaging result of their activity. Nonetheless, they can cause lesser or greater degrees of harm in the manner of a shingles eruption, bleeding ulcer, or disseminated cancer.

What Do Stealth Germs "Do"?

There are a number of ways stealth germs can do harm. One is by causing chronic organ scarring (cirrhosis of the liver due to hepatitis B or C, for example) as the result of years of long-standing and low-grade inflammation. Another, more deadly way stealth germs can do harm is in the eventual development of cancer; human papillomavirus, hepatitis viruses, and others have been implicated in different cancers.

Another danger of harboring a stealth infection is that the organisms can increase in numbers, reemerge, or disseminate throughout the body when the immune system is compromised, such as when undergoing cancer chemotherapy or in persons who have developed AIDS. It is well recognized that during chemotherapy, certain hidden infections can reemerge. For example, tuberculosis and coccidioidomycosis can suddenly emerge out of hiding. Toxoplasmosis in the eye and cytomegalovirus have also been shown to reactivate during chemotherapy. Certain viruses may be a factor in the rejection of transplanted kidneys when the body's immune system is suppressed to keep the body itself from rejecting the kidney. Therefore, in the case of persons who are about to undergo chemotherapy, it would be useful to know what if any stealth germs are hiding in their system. Nevertheless, detailed investigation to discover the presence of such stealth organisms in patients prior to starting chemotherapy is rarely undertaken.

Another way that a stealth organism can do its harm is by infecting others who come into intimate contact with the infected person. This hazard is well known in the case of herpesviruses, chlamydia, certain forms of hepatitis, and syphilis. Another especially hazardous situation may occur if a person harbors one (or more) infectious organism(s), and is exposed to yet another one, a so-called dual infection. For example, those who carry hepatitis C and then acquire schistosomiasis, or others who have Lyme disease then acquire other infections, or those who harbor herpesvirus then acquire HIV, or those exposed to malaria while also harboring HIV become significantly more ill than a person who has only one of the infections and not both.

Treatment Considerations

If you are found to harbor a stealth organism, shouldn't you receive prompt treatment to eradicate it? And will that treatment protect you against the damage it may be causing or might have already caused? This subject will also be discussed in more detail in chapter 7.

Even with proof of the causal relationship between a stealth germ and a disease, the benefits of treatment may not be obvious or guaranteed.

Some germs do their harm by acting in a hit-and-run fashion, striking and then disappearing from the host. During their temporary presence they may set in motion a cascade of immune reactions in the body and cause an ongoing or progressive disease condition even after the germs are long gone. These germs are like a trigger, setting off a sequence of events that produces the final or ongoing damage. It may do little good to try to eradicate the organism from the body when it is no longer present, or is still present but no longer needed for the response which continues on "autopilot." In such cases, the benefit, if any, of eradication or treatment needs to be verified by outcome studies.

Most physicians these days adhere to the principles of evidence-based medicine. Therefore, even if a stealth germ is present in the body, to fully convince physicians to treat asymptomatic carriers of stealth germs, it would be necessary to prove convincingly that the active presence of these organisms is what leads to later development of serious diseases such as cirrhosis of the liver, cancer of the cervix, cancer of the stomach, or a similar problem. Furthermore, it would have to be proven that eradicating the organism at a particular time actually alters such an outcome. Such proof is often extremely difficult or virtually impossible to achieve, and, for the most part, is currently not available. In the absence of incontrovertible proof, treatment becomes a matter of judgment, leading to the reluctance by many physicians to undertake active intervention in such cases.

However, as investigators and academics continue to look at the issue, attitudes of physicians regarding treatment are evolving. I personally believe that in many cases there is enough evidence even now to warrant taking action. Stealth germs can be thought of as criminals; when a criminal is on the loose, we cannot wait for absolute and final proof before we do something. In the case of stealth germs, we must take prudent protective measures and stop them in their tracks before they do more harm. Some may consider this an overreaction. Others may praise it as a reasonable proactive strategy. In various cases the true answer lies somewhere in between.

I believe that in many cases treatment is warranted, governed by the thoughtful and wise application of current knowledge. Some of these management decisions may not be fully supported by hard science. However, as I noted in the disclaimer, this book is not a scientific treatise; rather, it tries to explain approaches I have found useful in thirty years of medical practice and over 150,000 patient visits.

Stealth Infections of Regions of the Body

Individual stealth infections have various effects on different organ systems. However, aside from stealth germs, there are multitudes of other conditions and infections that can affect each of these organ systems. These can be found in comprehensive medical textbooks. By now it should be clear that this book is not aimed at discussing or uncovering every known disease, but is mainly intended to heighten your awareness, and to help steer you toward a correct diagnosis for some of the smoldering stealth infections I have chosen to highlight. (Please read the disclaimer, which appears at the front of the book.)

Fortunately the vast majority of you reading this book are probably healthy. If you have felt well all of your life, and don't remember being sick and have avoided exposure to those with possible infections, it is unlikely that you carry a stealth germ of consequence.

If you do have certain concerns, once again remember that there are many noninfectious conditions that may cause similar or even identical symptoms. Avoid the temptation to attribute all symptoms and problems to stealth germs. Additionally, when you discuss medical issues with friends and family, keep in mind that the same condition, infectious or noninfectious, will not affect everyone in the same way or to the same degree. One's symptoms or severity of illness depend on individual immunity, genetic makeup, and the coexistence of other infections or medical conditions. Some of these predispositions may cause an infectious agent to behave differently in one individual than it does in another. Many of the symptoms and findings described in this book and medical textbooks apply to the average patient. You, of course, may be a special case.

Read about conditions of the organ system where you think that you may have reason for concern. Afterward look up the suspected disease in a reputable source of medical information. Make sure that the textbook description of the suspected condition matches many or most of your symptoms, rather than just one or two. If you are still concerned, then see your doctor, and present your case in order to determine whether or not further action is necessary.

4. Stealth Infections of Body Regions

IN THIS SECTION, we will look at the human body region by region, and examine a few stealth infections associated with each particular region. Additionally, we will highlight some infections that may not truly be stealth infections, yet are sometimes overlooked or misdiagnosed. A few special issues, such as pregnancy, developmental problems, and animal-borne infections, are briefly discussed in chapter 5.

I have, where appropriate and possible, provided an illustrative "case in point" with references from the medical literature cited in the Notes at the end of the book. The descriptions are brief, general, and by no means complete. If you are curious about a particular condition, you should consult an up-to-date medical textbook or other peer-reviewed source for a complete description of the symptoms, diagnostic tests, and treatments that should be considered for each condition. Since diagnostic and treatment recommendations frequently change, consult your doctor for diagnosis and treatment for any suspected condition you may have. Some of the information provided here may change or rapidly become out of date. Use the information provided as a springboard to discussion and further inuqiry, rather than as a definitive guide to diagnosis and treatment.

We will examine possible stealth infection looking at the following bodily systems/regions and medical conditions:

Abdomen and Stomach (this region first, in recognition of *H. pylori*)

Arthritis and Joints

Blood and Lymphatic Diseases

Bone Infections

Bowels, Intestines, and Diarrhea

Brain and Psychiatric Conditions

Breast Disease

Cancers Linked to Stealth Infections

Ear Conditions

Endocrine System

Esophagus

Eye

Fatigue and Malaise

Feet and Ankles

Gynecologic and Pelvic Conditions

Head Symptoms

Heart and Cardiovascular Conditions

Kidneys and Stealth Infections

Liver and Hepatitis

Lung and Pulmonary Conditions

Male Genitals and Prostate

Mouth and Throat

Muscles

Neurological and Nervous Conditions

Nose and Sinuses

Obesity and Stealth Germs

Stealth Infections and the Skin

Urinary Tract and Bladder Conditions

After discussing the conditions of these organ systems we will proceed to look at considerations involved in the treatment and prevention of these conditions, and look ahead to the future.

Abdomen and Stomach (Gastrointestinal System)

See also sections on Bowels Intestines and Diarrhea, and Esophagus.

There are many conditions of the gastrointestinal system, which can cause a variety of symptoms or problems. Acid indigestion, gassiness, and sensitive stomach are frequently encountered symptoms. Many cases are not related to stealth infections, but some are due to treatable infections that should be considered.

Ulcer Bacteria Causing Ulcers

Symptom: sensitive stomach, acid indigestion, stomachaches, prior stomach ulcer

Descriptive Diagnosis: stomach ulcer, gastritis, acid indigestion

Actual Diagnosis: stomach infection caused by *H. pylori*

Stealth Infection: Helicobacter pylori

Tests to Consider: blood test, stool test, and other tests for *H. pylori*

Potential Treatment: antibiotics, concurrently with an acid suppressant

Case in Point: Stomach ulcers are the most notable result of harboring ulcer bacteria. However, even in the presence of this bacteria, ulcers will often improve when treated with strong acid-suppressant medicines. In the presence of *H. pylori*, however, the stomach is more sensitive than usual to irritants, including aspirin, anti-inflammatory medicines, coffee, alcohol, and black pepper and other substances. Anyone with a history of ulcers who has not been tested previously should have a test for infection with *H. pylori*. Some patients will show evidence of prior exposure, but no active infection is found. However, even if you have been treated previously, you could relapse or reacquire the infection.

Ulcer Bacteria Causing Chronically Sensitive Stomach

Symptom: chronic acid indigestion and chronically sensitive stomach, easily irritated by coffee, alcohol, aspirin, anti-inflammatories or other substances

Descriptive Diagnosis: chronic acid indigestion, chronic gastritis, pyrosis, gastroesophageal reflux disease (GERD)

Actual Diagnosis: Helicobacter pylori stomach infection

Stealth Infection: H. pylori

Tests to Consider: blood test, stool test, and other tests for *H. pylori*

Potential Treatment: antibiotics, concurrently with acid suppressant

Case in Point: Patients with a long-standing sensitive stomach are often told they have chronic gastritis, and that they should eliminate coffee, alcohol, aspirin, black pepper, and other stomach irritants. However, stomach sensitivity persists even if they take antacids. When tested, they are found to have *H. pylori* colonization, even though they never had a proven ulcer. Other times, ingested chemicals or foodstuffs may be the culprit, rather than infection. However, substances generally irritating to the stomach will be much more so in a person whose stomach is already inflamed by infection.

Chronically "Gassy Stomach" due to Giardia

Symptom: long-standing upper stomach bloating, gassiness, sensitive stomach, some acid indigestion

Descriptive Diagnosis: chronic gastritis, irritable bowel syndrome, gassiness

Actual Diagnosis: giardiasis

Stealth Infection: Giardia lamblia

Tests to Consider: stool or other tests for Giardia

Potential Treatment: various specific antibiotics

Case in Point: Giardia lamblia is an organism frequently found in stream and well water. Campers or others who drink contaminated water will ingest the organism, which colonizes the duodenum, the gastrointestinal passage that exits from the stomach. Colonization usually causes persistent, low-grade upper abdominal gas symptoms, sensitive stomach, and looser stools than usual. Those who have secretory IgA deficiency in the stomach lining or duodenum are especially likely to acquire *Giardia lamblia.* Untreated, colonization may persist for years. Persons are often told they have incurable irritable bowel syndrome, and the infection is overlooked, yet symptoms resolve with proper treatment.

Persistent Right Upper Abdominal Pain in Women, Related to Pelvic Infection

Symptom: persistent right upper abdominal pain in a young woman, which is not responsive to medicines taken for indigestion; there may or may not be pelvic symptoms

Descriptive Diagnosis: stomach pain of unknown source, irritable bowel syndrome, hepatic flexure syndrome, stomach gas, gallbladder problems

Actual Diagnosis: Fitz-Hugh–Curtis syndrome

Stealth Infection: chlamydia or other pelvic bacteria

Tests to Consider: pelvic examination and culture for chlamydia; consider empiric treatment with appropriate antibiotics

Potential Treatment: antibiotics used for treating pelvic infections

Case in Point: This problem may arise in a young, sexually active woman. She may or may not have significant pelvic symptoms, but may have been diagnosed previously with a vaginal infection or other pelvic infection and received treatment. She develops persistent right upper abdominal pains, which feel like a "stitch in the side." It is not related to eating or drinking, or emptying the bladder or moving the bowels. It does not respond to conventional medicines such as antacids. She may have been told that it was due to gas, irritable bowel syndrome, hepatic flexure syndrome, and may have been tested for gallstones. Ultrasound and CT scan results are negative. The possibility that her symptoms indicate Fitz-Hugh–Curtis syndrome caused by bacteria spreading up from the pelvis is sometimes missed, except by careful diagnosticians.

Yeast (Candida) Colonization of the Stomach in Diabetics or in Persons Taking Prednisone or Other Corticosteroids

Symptom: sensitive stomach in person with long-standing diabetes or other conditions or treatments, such as prednisone, which suppress the immune system

Descriptive Diagnosis: acid indigestion, chronic gastritis, pyrosis, gastroesophageal reflux disease (GERD)

Actual Diagnosis: yeast infection of stomach

Stealth Infection: *Candida albicans*

Tests to Consider: scope test of the stomach and esophagus to look for yeast; may consider empiric treatment with antiyeast medicines

Potential Treatment: antiyeast medicine in liquid or tablet form

Case in Point: Persons taking antibiotics, or on medicines such as prednisone or immune suppressants, and the elderly or diabetics, are at risk for yeast infections. The mouth, esophagus, and stomach can become overrun by yeast, as well as the vaginal area in women. Yeast infection of the stomach or the esophagus may be overlooked because these surfaces are not visible. Instead, the stomach symptoms may be treated with antacid preparations, which are not effective. In these patients, brief empiric treatment with an antiyeast medicine sometimes yields remarkable and prompt improvement of stomach symptoms previously not responsive to the usual stomach therapies.

Arthritis and Joints

See also section on Bone Infections.

Lyme disease is a rheumatologic condition caused by a smoldering, hard-to-diagnose infection. The sexually transmitted infection gonorrhea can cause inflamed joints. Most rheumatologic conditions are not directly due to active smoldering infections. However, conditions such as Reiter's syndrome and possibly rheumatoid arthritis may be triggered by an infection.

Unusual joint infections may occur in persons who are on immune suppressants or cancer chemotherapy. Lurking stealth infections, such as tuberculosis, or the fungal spores of coccidioidomycosis (valley fever), that have been dormant in the body for decades, can re-emerge out of hiding and show up suddenly in the form of an inflamed joint.

Arthritis and Other Symptoms Caused by Lyme Disease

Symptom: joint aches and pains beginning a few weeks following a skin rash that followed a tick bite; also, fatigue and nervous system symptoms, such as mental fatigue, headaches, or memory problems

Descriptive Diagnosis: arthritis, chronic fatigue, fibromyalgia

Actual Diagnosis: Lyme disease

Stealth Infection: Borrelia burgdorferi

Tests to Consider: antibody or other tests specific for Lyme disease

Potential Treatment: antibiotics specific for Lyme disease

Case in Point: Named after the town of Lyme, Connecticut, where the condition first came to attention, the stealth germ that causes the condition is transmitted by deer ticks. The infection affects mostly joints, but may spread to the central nervous system/brain and the heart. The initial symptom is a patchy skin rash (erythema chronicum migrans), which soon disappears without treatment. The rash is followed within several days to weeks by recurrent, scattered joint pains. Later brain symptoms, heart symptoms, and fatigue and malaise usually develop. Antibiotics given too late may not always be helpful.

Reiter's Syndrome (Reactive Arthritis) Triggered by Bowel or Sexually Transmitted Infections

Symptom: joint aches and pains associated with urinary and prostate symptoms in men, mostly in those with genetic susceptibility indicated by the HLA–B27 marker

Descriptive Diagnosis: arthritis or prostate infection

Actual Diagnosis: Reiter's syndrome, reactive arthritis

Stealth Infection: salmonella, *Chlamydia trachomatis*

Tests to Consider: HLA–B27 test; also, test for chlamydia and/or sal-monella

Potential Treatment: early treatment of infection with various antibi-otics

Case in Point: Patients with so-called reactive arthritis usually develop joint aches and pains ten to thirty days after a bowel infection with diarrhea, or a sexually transmitted infection that had caused urinary or prostate symptoms. Patients, mostly men, develop miscellaneous joint aches and pains and certain other inflammatory symptoms that may affect the eyes. Some have recurrent or persistent episodes of discomfort on urination. Active infection or a carrier state of the above organisms needs to be tested. If found, treatment of chronic prostatitis or the salmonella carrier state is warranted. Early treatment of all infections in persons who carry the HLA–B27 susceptibility gene is generally advised.

Rheumatoid Arthritis Triggered by Viral Infection in Susceptible Individuals

Symptom: usual symptoms of rheumatoid arthritis (RA) including inflammation and swelling of multiple joints symmetrically through-out the body

Descriptive Diagnosis: rheumatoid arthritis

Actual Diagnosis: rheumatoid arthritis

Stealth Infection: RA–1 parvovirus suspected as a trigger

Tests to Consider: no common test is used for this potential infectious trigger

Potential Treatment: doxycycline is partially effective in early cases of RA, though it does not treat the virus

Case in Point: Rheumatoid arthritis in its very early stages responds to a small extent to the antibiotic doxycycline, but the benefit is believed to be due to the medicine's anti-inflammatory effect, rather than its anti-infective effect. There is strong suspicion that rheumatoid arthritis is an overreaction of the body's immune system to a hit-and-run viral infection, possibly the RA-1 parvovirus. Even if treatment were available, it would be unlikely to reverse the already-triggered immune reaction. Rheumatoid arthritis at this time is treated with conventional treatments outlined in medical textbooks, including anti-inflammatories, immune system suppressants, and tumor necrosis factor inhibitors.

Arthritis Due to Gonorrhea

Symptom: joint pains and swelling with fever and urinary or pelvic discharge suggestive of sexually transmitted infection

Descriptive Diagnosis: infected joint or arthritis due to infection

Actual Diagnosis: gonorrheal joint infection

Stealth Infection: Neisseria gonorrhoeae (gonorrhea)

Tests to Consider: culture of urethra in men, pelvis in women, culture joint fluid

Potential Treatment: antibiotics customarily used to treat gonorrhea

Case in Point: In Reiter's syndrome, sexually transmitted or other infections can trigger so-called reactive arthritis, causing inflammation of the joints, though the infectious organism itself is not in the joint. In contrast, in cases of gonorrhea, the organism spreads through the bloodstream and directly infects various joints. A person may carry gonorrhea for a while before the joint symptoms appear.

Reactivated Tuberculosis Causing Arthritis

Symptom: inflamed, painful joint in person on prednisone or immunosuppressive or cancer chemotherapy, who years earlier may have had exposure to tuberculosis

Descriptive Diagnosis: inflammatory arthritis of a single joint, attributed to gout or rheumatoid arthritis

Actual Diagnosis: joint infection with tuberculosis

Stealth Infection: *Mycobacterium tuberculosis* (tuberculosis)

Tests to Consider: biopsy and culture of the inflamed joint

Potential Treatment: usual antituberculous antibiotics

Case in Point: An older patient developed cancer and received chemotherapy treatment. As a child, he had been exposed to tuberculosis—his mother died of the infection. He himself never had signs of active TB. While being treated for cancer, he developed a couple of inflamed and swollen joints that continued off and on for a few months. Gout was considered as a possible cause, since the swollen joint improved temporarily with strong anti-inflammatories, the usual therapy for gout. Rheumatoid arthritis was also considered. When the inflamed joint kept relapsing, a biopsy was performed, and the tuberculosis organism was found in the joint.

Reactivated Infection with Coccidioidomycosis Causing Arthritis

Symptom: inflamed, painful joint in person on prednisone, immunosuppressive drugs, or cancer chemotherapy, who may have granulomas on X-rays

Descriptive Diagnosis: inflammatory arthritis of single joint, attributed to gout or rheumatoid arthritis

Actual Diagnosis: joint infection with coccidioidomycosis

Stealth Infection: *Coccidioides immitis*

Tests to Consider: culture and biopsy of the inflamed joint

Potential Treatment: antifungal medication

Case in Point: A patient had a long history of asthma, which was periodically treated with prednisone. He later developed rheumatoid arthritis, and over many years was treated with prednisone and other medicines that suppress the immune system. While on treatment, he developed one exceptionally swollen joint in his hand. It did not respond to increasing the dose of his rheumatoid arthritis medication. The joint was biopsied and was found to be infected with *Coccidioides immitis*, the fungal organism that causes coccidioidomycosis, or valley fever. The joint improved after treatment with the appropriate antifungal medication.

Orthopedic Infections and Sciatica Caused by Acne Bacteria

Symptom: infection of joints repaired with joint implants through orthopedic surgery and possibly sciatica

Descriptive Diagnosis: infected joint implant, inflammatory sciatica

Actual Diagnosis: infected joint implant or sciatica caused by a specific infection

Stealth Infection: *Propionibacterium acnes* (acne bacteria) (suspected, but not proven)

Tests to Consider: none for those with sciatica; culture of the infected joint for those with joint infection

Potential Treatment: antibiotics specific for the suspected infection

Case in Point: Postoperative infection of prosthetic joints with skin organisms occurs, mostly with staphylococcus. However, when staph does not grow from the inflamed joint, infection with the acne bacteria *Propionibacterium* should be considered. Though the evidence is preliminary, the role of this organism in prosthetic joint implant infections and prosthesis failure, as well as sciatica, is being investigated.

Reactive Arthritis After Unnamed Virus Exposure

Symptom: acute or persistent arthritis

Descriptive Diagnosis: arthritis, flu syndrome

Actual Diagnosis: reactive arthritis caused by parvovirus

Stealth Infection: parvovirus B19

Tests to Consider: serum tests available, but not commonly used

Potential Treatment: no specific treatment available

Case in Point: A 30-year-old woman had acute swelling of her hands and wrists two weeks after her son had fifth disease ("slapped cheek" syndrome), even though she had no particular signs of illness other than the joint symptoms. Her problem persisted for several weeks. There is high incidence of exposure to parvovirus among schoolteachers who are in contact with children. Parvovirus infection can occasionally mimic the symptoms of rheumatoid arthritis.

Lupus (Systemic Lupus Erythematosus) Triggered by Stealth Infection

Symptom: usual symptoms of lupus, including joint pains and swelling, occasionally with fever and skin symptoms

Descriptive Diagnosis: arthritis due to lupus

Actual Diagnosis: systemic lupus erythematosus

Stealth Infection: Lupus develops in part due to errors made by Toll-like receptors (TLRs) in the body, which are normally able to distinguish between the self and microbes which are not members of the normal flora. The microbes parvovirus B19 and *Mycoplasma penetrans* have been implicated as possible triggers of the abnormal reaction, which then leads to the symptoms of lupus.

Tests to Consider: no specific test recommended for the infectious trigger

Potential Treatment: no specific treatment for the infectious trigger, though medicines against mycoplasma are available.

Case in Point: In patients with typical presentation of lupus, an infectious trigger should be considered. If a treatable one is found in the patient's system, treatment may be considered, though it may not help. Treatable organisms harbored by many persons with or without lupus are mycoplasma, chlamydia, and herpesviruses, including cytomegalovirus. One should always be on the lookout for dual conditions, namely the presence of more than one infection, or the carrier state of more than one infection, at the same time. Each should be diagnosed and treated properly.

Blood and Lymphatic Diseases

See also section on Fatigue and Malaise.

Certain stealth infections do not confine themselves to a specific location in the body. Instead, they may circulate in the blood, or spread through the lymphatic system. These organisms may cause general symptoms such as fatigue, malaise, or symptoms that are scattered throughout the body and its various organ systems. Historically, the sexually transmitted infection syphilis, which can work in this way, was called the "great masquerader" for its ability to mimic other conditions. The most notorious blood-borne stealth infection today is the human immunodeficiency virus (HIV) which may circulate for years throughout the body before it causes significant symptoms and evolves into acquired immunodeficiency syndrome, or AIDS. Patients with early HIV symptoms are sometimes initially diagnosed as having chronic fatigue syndrome or fibromyalgia.

Syphilis, the "Great Masquerader," Causing Problems Throughout the Body

Symptom: rash and enlarged lymph nodes that eventually disappear; years may pass without symptoms, eventually followed by slowly evolving vascular conditions, problems with memory, concentration, or balance

Descriptive Diagnosis: early—viral syndrome; late—vasculitis, dementia

Actual Diagnosis: primary, secondary, and tertiary syphilis

Stealth Infection: *Treponema pallidum* (syphilis)

Tests to Consider: blood tests and spinal fluid tests for syphilis

Potential Treatment: usual antibiotics for the infection

Case in Point: An elderly patient developed progressive memory and concentration problems that were diagnosed as dementia. During evaluation, a routine screening blood test was positive for syphilis. The patient was aware that their spouse, now deceased, had had an extramarital affair, but neither partner was tested for exposure to this sexually transmitted disease. A spinal fluid examination was done, and there was evidence of active syphilis infection in the spinal fluid.

Human Immunodeficiency Virus (HIV) Causing AIDS and Complications

Symptom: transient flu-like illness, followed by disappearance of the symptoms, except for a low-grade malaise; eventually fevers, recurrent infections, and complications develop due to immune deficiency

Descriptive Diagnosis: early, flu syndrome; later, chronic fatigue

Actual Diagnosis: HIV carrier state, AIDS

Stealth Infection: human immunodeficiency virus (HIV)

Tests to Consider: HIV test

Potential Treatment: usual antiviral treatment for HIV/AIDS

Case in Point: HIV is a classic stealth infection, causing low-grade flu-like symptoms as it enters the body. Sometimes it causes hardly any symptoms at all. It continues to spread through the body with minimal symptoms for years. Over time, it damages part of the immune system and predisposes the infected individual to various infections and cancers.

Leukemia Caused by Viral Infection

Symptom: fatigue, malaise, abnormal blood test

Descriptive Diagnosis: adult T-cell leukemia

Actual Diagnosis: leukemia due to virus infection

Stealth Infection: human T-cell lymphotropic virus type I (HTLV-I)

Tests to Consider: blood test for the virus

Potential Treatment: no treatment for the virus; leukemia treated with chemotherapy

Case in Point: A number of viruses are known to cause leukemia in animals. Most cases of leukemia in adults have not yet been conclusively linked to viruses. Adult T-cell leukemia is an uncommon type of leukemia, occurring in certain areas of the world such as southern Japan and the Caribbean. It has been linked to the so-called human T-cell lymphotropic virus type I.

Reactivation of Malaria Acquired Abroad

Symptom: persistent nighttime fevers, chills, and sweats several years after exposure to malaria or travel to malaria-infested regions or countries

Descriptive Diagnosis: fever of unknown origin (FUO)

Actual Diagnosis: malaria

Stealth Infection: *Plasmodium ovale*

Tests to Consider: "thick and thin smear" blood test for malaria

Potential Treatment: specific antimalarial antibiotics

Case in Point: A person who lived most of his life in Africa was treated six years earlier for probable malaria. About that time he moved to the United States, and for the next several years he was symptom-free. At one point, he developed persistent nighttime fevers and chills. After testing, his condition was found to be due to recurrence of malaria, which had been dormant for several years. Malaria infection typically develops one month after initial exposure. In rare cases, it can remain as a stealth germ in the bloodstream and reemerge and cause relapse of symptoms years later.

West Nile Virus Passed on Through Blood Transfusion

Symptom: fever subsequent to blood transfusion

Descriptive Diagnosis: transfusion reaction, viral infection

Actual Diagnosis: West Nile virus infection

Stealth Infection: West Nile virus

Tests to Consider: serum test for the virus

Potential Treatment: none

Case in Point: Eighty percent of cases of West Nile virus infection cause little or no symptoms in the infected person. However, even if there are no symptoms, a person may have the virus actively circulating in their blood for a period of time after exposure. If he or she donates blood during that time, the person receiving the blood transfusion may develop symptoms and illness characteristic of the West Nile virus infection.

Cytomegalovirus Causing Frailty and Cognitive Decline in the Elderly, or Relapsing Fatigue in Younger Persons, Especially in Immunocompromised Individuals

Symptom: recurrent low-grade malaise, fatigue, sometimes accompanied lymphadenopathy

Descriptive Diagnosis: chronic fatigue, frailty in the elderly

Actual Diagnosis: cytomegalovirus infection

Stealth Infection: cytomegalovirus (CMV)

Tests to Consider: IgM and IgG serology specific for CMV, or urine culture for cytomegalovirus while symptoms are active

Potential Treatment: antiviral medication available

Case in Point: Recent reports indicate an association between frailty and cognitive decline in the elderly and prior exposure to this virus. Cytomegalovirus is a member of the human herpesvirus family, and may "cycle" in persons who have weakened immunity. The role of cytomegalovirus in persons with chronic fatigue syndrome has been considered. There may be some persons with periodic relapsing fatigue whose symptoms may be due to this organism. In persons receiving chemotherapy, or those with AIDS, serious flare-up of a lurking cytomegalovirus infection may occur, and treatment with antiviral medication is available and warranted. Medical problems caused by cytomegalovirus may be underdiagnosed, due to the mistaken belief that treatment is not available.

Lyme Disease Causing Various Symptoms

Symptom: fatigue, arthritis, neurological symptoms

Descriptive Diagnosis: chronic fatigue, arthritis

Actual Diagnosis: Lyme disease

Stealth Infection: Borrelia burgdorferi

Tests to Consider: various blood tests for Lyme disease

Potential Treatment: antibiotics

Case in Point: Already described in the section under arthritis, Lyme disease can cause a variety of nonspecific symptoms while it circulates in the bloodstream. Because of the absence of fever, chills, and inflammation, and the gradual and protracted symptomatology, the presence of an active infection may not be considered.

Immune Thrombocytopenic Purpura Blood Disorder Linked to H. pylori

Symptom: rapidly spreading tiny red spots on legs and elsewhere on the skin

Descriptive Diagnosis: immune thrombocytopenic purpura (ITP)

Actual Diagnosis: ITP triggered by underlying infection

Stealth Infection: Helicobacter pylori (suspected)

Tests to Consider: blood and stool test for H. pylori

Potential Treatment: usual treatment for ITP and also for H. pylori

Case in Point: There are reports that patients who develop a blood disorder associated with very low blood platelet counts, called immune thrombocytopenic purpura often have evidence of infection with *H. pylori*. Some of the patients treated with antibiotics aimed at eradicating the *H. pylori* infection show improvement of the low platelet counts that characterize this condition.

Blood Transfusions Transmitting Various Infections

Symptom: fever, fatigue, arthritis, neurological symptoms soon after receiving blood transfusion

Descriptive Diagnosis: blood transfusion reaction

Actual Diagnosis: infection acquired from blood transfusion

Stealth Infection: gram-positive and gram-negative bacteria, Human herpesvirus type 8, cytomegalovirus, Creutzfeldt-Jakob prion

Tests to Consider: blood cultures, serology tests

Potential Treatment: antibiotics, antivirals

Case in Point: Even though the blood supply is very carefully screened for infectious organisms, it is impossible to test for every known virus or other organism that may be in the donor's system. Occasionally unexpected organisms such as the ones noted above may be present in the donor blood, and be the cause of a "transfusion reaction." Persons who have new-onset unusual symptoms, including symptoms similar to those noted above following a blood transfusion, should undergo a careful search for possible infection transmitted through the transfused blood.

Subacute Bacterial Endocarditis due to Various Infectious Organisms

Symptom: malaise, low-grade fevers

Descriptive Diagnosis: chronic fatigue, fever of unknown origin (FUO)

Actual Diagnosis: subacute bacterial endocarditis

Stealth Infection: streptococci, *Brucella* species, *Coxiella burnetii*, *Haemophilus* bacteria; rarely, fungi or other bacteria

Tests to Consider: blood cultures; culture of the nose, urine; serology tests

Potential Treatment: antibiotics

Case in Point: Subacute bacterial endocarditis is also one of the great mimickers. It may cause a variety of nonspecific symptoms and evolve over weeks or several months, with fatigue and weakness, some sweats, vague aches and pains, and some weight loss. Due to the lack of high fevers or chills, an infection may not be suspected until symptoms persist or become considerably worse.

Severe Anemia due to Acquired Pure Red Cell Aplasia Caused by Infections

Symptom: malaise, fatigue due to anemia

Descriptive Diagnosis: severe anemia due to acquired pure red cell aplasia

Actual Diagnosis: same, due to infection

Stealth Infection: parvovirus B19, mumps, hepatitis, Epstein–Barr virus, HIV (rarely)

Tests to Consider: various tests for the above infectious

Potential Treatment: some of the above infections are treatable with anti-infectives

Case in Point: Severe anemia not found to be due to any nutritional deficiencies or blood loss is sometimes diagnosed to be the condition called acquired pure red cell aplasia. There is evidence that the infections listed above can be the cause of this condition.

Bone Infections

See also section describing arthritis and joint problems.

Infections that invade noninjured bones are not very common. Osteomyelitis is the most notable such condition. Staphylococcus harbored in a person's nose, acting as a stealth germ, can spread through the blood and "seed" certain bones, often in the spine. Rarely, persons who harbor tuberculosis develop tuberculous osteomyelitis in the spine, also known as Pott's disease. See also the discussion of infected artificial joints described previously.

Osteomyelitis Caused by Staphylococcus ("Staph") Bacteria Harbored in the Nose

Symptom: severe unremitting back pain due to bone infection

Descriptive Diagnosis: osteomyelitis of bone in the spine

Actual Diagnosis: osteomyelitis with *Staphylococcus aureus*

Stealth Infection: *Staphylococcus aureus* harbored in the nose

Tests to Consider: culture nose for staph in addition to cultures of infected material obtained from the spine

Potential Treatment: antistaph antibiotics, including measures to eradicate staph from nose to reduce the likelihood of future recurrences

Case in Point: A middle-aged, otherwise healthy man developed rapidly progressive severe pain in his back. X-rays suggested infectious osteomyelitis of the spine. The patient had had chronic nasal congestion for years, with a crusty discharge and occasional sores inside the nasal passages, but was otherwise healthy. A nose culture confirmed the presence of *Staphylococcus aureus*, also isolated from the infected bone in his spine. No other obvious source of staph bacteria was found on his body.

Osteomyelitis from Reactivated Tuberculosis That Spread Through the Bloodstream

Symptom: severe unremitting back pain due to bone infection

Descriptive Diagnosis: osteomyelitis of vertebra

Actual Diagnosis: Pott's disease of the spine caused by tuberculosis organism

Stealth Infection: Mycobacterium tuberculosis

Tests to Consider: culture material obtained from the spine for so-called acid-fast bacteria, in addition to usual bacterial cultures

Potential Treatment: antituberculous antibiotics

Case in Point: Person with no prior history of active tuberculosis, but history of a granuloma on an old chest X-ray and positive TB skin test, developed progressive severe upper back pain along with some low-grade fevers. X-ray results suggested osteomyelitis. Biopsy of the infected vertebra confirmed the presence of tuberculosis organisms.

Bowel, Intestines, and Diarrhea

See also section on Abdomen and Stomach.

There are numerous noninfectious conditions that cause abdominal symptoms such as gassiness, loose bowels, abdominal discomfort, and abdominal pains. Some of these are food sensitivites, including to milk and dairy products in those with lactose intolerance; to wheat in persons with gluten sensitive enteropathy (celiac disease); to carbonated beverages, beer, excessive doses of vitamin C, and many other supplements or medicines. Chronic constipation can also cause bloating and discomfort. When no particular cause is found, physicians often label such symptoms irritable bowel syndrome. There are also many infections that cause obvious acute gastrointestinal illnesses characterized by acute diarrhea, pain, vomiting, and fever. These are usually correctly attributed to infection and properly treated.

Treatable stealth organisms can take up long-term residence in the bowels, and can cause ongoing, low-grade, smoldering symptoms, which are often misattributed to "noncurable" irritable bowel syndrome or colitis. In many cases, an infection can be diagnosed, and a well-chosen antibiotic can substantially improve and sometimes cure these symptoms. In other cases, where there is an acquired imbalance of the normal flora, probiotics may be helpful.

Irritable Bowel Syndrome Due to Giardia

Symptom: chronic gassy stomach and loose bowels

Descriptive Diagnosis: irritable bowel syndrome

Actual Diagnosis: giardiasis

Stealth Infection: Giardia lamblia

Tests to Consider: stool and other tests for Giardia

Potential Treatment: antibiotics specific for Giardia

Case in Point: Giardia lamblia is a very common organism, which lives in well or stream water. When ingested through drinking contaminated water, or eating food washed with contaminated water, Giardia colonizes the duodenum, and can cause ongoing low-grade gassy and loose bowels, which is often attributed to irritable bowel syndrome and treated with various stomach remedies. When the organism is correctly identified and treated with the correct antibiotic, the symptoms are often much improved or cured.

Irritable Bowel Syndrome Due to Blastocystis

Symptom: chronic gassy bowels and loose stools

Descriptive Diagnosis: irritable bowel syndrome

Actual Diagnosis: *Blastocystis* infestation

Stealth Infection: *Blastocystis hominis*

Tests to Consider: stools for ova and parasites

Potential Treatment: antibiotics specific for *Blastocystis*

Case in Point: This organism may be found in the bowels of travelers to underdeveloped countries who return home with loose stools, gassiness, and other nonspecific bowel symptoms, which were not present before the trip. Often they are told that they have irritable bowel syndrome. Stool testing may reveal *Blastocystis*. Whether *Blastocystis* is the sole cause of all of their symptoms is often questioned. However, in many cases, after antibiotic treatment the bowels return to their former condition.

Irritable Bowel Syndrome Due to Entamoeba coli

Symptom: chronic gassy bowels and loose stools that develop after travel abroad

Descriptive Diagnosis: irritable bowel syndrome

Actual Diagnosis: *Entamoeba coli* infestation

Stealth Infection: *Entamoeba coli*

Tests to Consider: stool for ova and parasites

Potential Treatment: medicines used for ameba

Case in Point: A person who has traveled abroad may return with on a stool test. This organism is generally believed to be a "harmless" distant cousin of *Entamoeba histolytica*, the cause of amebiasis. Because it's considered nonpathogenic, some doctors won't treat it. However, its presence is usually a sign that the person was exposed to food or water contaminated with human fecal material, which may have also contained other organisms. Search for other organisms causing dual infection and treatment with medicines aimed at these organisms should be considered.

Persistent Diarrhea Following Antibiotic Use

Symptom: persistent, sometimes recurrent significant diarrhea following antibiotic use

Descriptive Diagnosis: antibiotic-related diarrhea

Actual Diagnosis: *Clostridium difficile* enterocolitis

Stealth Infection: *Clostridium difficile*

Tests to Consider: stool tests for *C. difficile* (toxin)

Potential Treatment: antibiotics specific for *C. difficile*

Case in Point: Some antibiotics, such as ampicillin, commonly cause diarrhea due to direct medication effect. *"C. diff"* is a frequent cause of persistent significant diarrhea and bowel symptoms that develop following treatment with certain antibiotics for infections elsewhere in the body. The toxin produced by the organism is primarily responsible for causing the diarrhea. Resistance of *C. difficile* to traditionally used antibiotics is an increasing problem. Even if you were given appropriate treatment for this condition, but have recurrent or persistent symptoms, you should be retested and treated appropriately. Another cause of diarrhea following antibiotic use could be yeast overgrowth.

Persistent Abdominal Bloating or Diarrhea Due to Bacterial Overgrowth of Small Intestine

Symptom: persistent diarrhea or altered bowel pattern in persons with conditions causing slow bowel transit in the small intestine

Descriptive Diagnosis: irritable bowel syndrome, chronic diarrhea of unknown source, colitis

Actual Diagnosis: bacterial overgrowth of small intestine

Stealth Infection: various bowel bacteria

Tests to Consider: no reliable test.

Potential Treatment: consider empiric trial of antibiotics in suspected cases

Case in Point: Bacterial overgrowth of small intestine is a condition that is not usually considered in cases of persistent diarrhea. Nevertheless, if bacteria invade the normally sterile small intestine, the result can be diarrhea and malabsorption of foods. This can happen in persons with abnormally slow propulsion in the intestines, such as in scleroderma or diabetes. In such cases the last part of the small intestine, the jejunum, becomes colonized with bacteria usually confined to the colon. Persistent diarrhea due to this problem improves when antibiotics are given to clear the bacteria from the small intestine.

Chronic Diarrhea and Weight Loss Due to Whipple's Disease

Symptom: chronic diarrhea and weight loss

Descriptive Diagnosis: irritable bowel syndrome, colitis

Actual Diagnosis: Whipple's disease

Stealth Infection: *Tropheryma whippelii*

Tests to Consider: small bowel biopsy

Potential Treatment: various antibiotics

Case in Point: Tropheryma whippelii is a little-known organism, which causes a condition called Whipple's disease. The symptoms of Whipple's disease are weight loss and loose bowels. Other symptoms, including neurological signs suggestive of early dementia, may evolve. The bacteria that cause this condition reside in the small intestine, and cannot be cultured on conventional stool tests. Unless the condition is suspected, it will be overlooked. Proof of the infection is obtained only if the small bowel is biopsied, and treatment with antibiotics will cure the condition.

Inflammatory Bowel Disease Possibly Due to Infection

Symptom: unremitting diarrhea, sometimes bloody

Descriptive Diagnosis: inflammatory bowel disease, ulcerative colitis, Crohn's disease

Actual Diagnosis: infectious colitis

Stealth Infection: Blastocystis hominis, amoeba, possibly other parasites

Tests to Consider: stool tests for ova and parasites

Potential Treatment: treat specific organism, if found; consider empiric treatment with metronidazole, which has been reported to improve the symptoms in some individuals with inflammatory bowel disease

Case in Point: On rare occasion, a person diagnosed with inflammatory bowel disease may have an infection of the bowel with a parasite or amoeba. Even if the organisms found on stool testing are considered to be nonpathogenic, treatment may be useful. The presence of nonpathogenic parasites or amoebas (such as *Blastocystis hominis* or *Entamoeba coli*) may indicate that contaminated food was ingested, which may have harbored other organisms that don't easily show up on stool tests. There are reports that some cases of inflammatory bowel disease improve in part when treated with antibiotics such as metronidazole. Even if stool tests do not show a particular infectious organism, a course of such antibiotics may be worthwhile in persons newly diagnosed with inflammatory bowel disease. Certain probiotics may be useful in cases of inflammatory bowel disease.

Proctitis Due to Sexually Transmitted Diseases

Symptom: persistent rectal irritation and feeling of rectal urgency, mucous discharge, possibly bloody; these symptoms are often attributed to hemorrhoids or fissures

Descriptive Diagnosis: proctitis, anal fissures, hemorrhoids

Actual Diagnosis: infectious proctitis

Stealth Infection: *Neisseria gonorrhoeae* (gonorrhea) and/or chlamydia, Lymphogranuloma venereum

Tests to Consider: sigmoidoscopy with cultures of rectum

Potential Treatment: various antibiotics

Case in Point: Proctitis due to such infections usually happens in sexually active persons who may have had exposure of the rectal area to sexually transmissible infections. *Neisseria gonorrhoeae* and chlamydia can both cause proctitis. If untreated, these organisms can cause further problems such as arthritis from disseminated gonorrhea, and may be transmitted to other sexual partners. Human papillomavirus may also be transmitted to the rectum, and the skin of the anal canal can also be infected by fungus and yeast, which cause chronic irritation similar to hemorrhoidal symptoms.

Salmonella (Typhoid) Carrier State May Infect Others

Symptom: persistent nonspecific stomachaches after eating contaminated food

Descriptive Diagnosis: irritable bowel syndrome, acid indigestion

Actual Diagnosis: salmonella carrier state

Stealth Infection: salmonella bacteria

Tests to Consider: febrile agglutinins, stool culture

Potential Treatment: antibiotics

Case in Point: A well-known historical case of salmonella acting as a stealth germ is the historic case of Typhoid Mary. Mary Mallon, a cook for a well-to-do family in New York around 1900 allegedly had no symptoms, yet carried the salmonella/typhoid organism and infected numerous persons in the household. Those interested in how a person may carry salmonella with minimal or no symptoms, yet be contagious to others, should read her interesting story. Salmonella carrier state may cause persons with certain predispositions to develop seemingly unrelated conditions, such as Reiter's syndrome.

Reiter's Syndrome Triggered by Bowel Infection

Symptom: diarrhea, abdominal pains, followed by joint pains

Descriptive Diagnosis: gastroenteritis, arthritis, possible Reiter's syndrome

Actual Diagnosis: Reiter's syndrome triggered by gastrointestinal infection

Stealth Infection: *Campylobacter jejuni* or *Shigella*

Tests to Consider: stool tests

Potential Treatment: antibiotics specific for the above organisms

Case in Point: This condition was described in more detail in section under Arthritis and Joints.

Brain and Psychiatric Conditions

See also sections on Neurological and Nervous Conditions, on Head Symptoms, and on Fatigue and Malaise.

Meningitis and encephalitis are usually severe in their symptoms, causing severe headache, confusion, sometimes obtundation and even seizures. However, some mild cases of these infections can present with minimal, subclinical symptoms, which are misattributed to noninfectious causes.

Chronic, slowly evolving brain problems are not often attributed to infections. Recent evidence indicates that certain cases of dementia, possibly schizophrenia, and even some seizure disorders may be related to exposure to, or rarely active infection with, certain stealth germs.

Dementia Caused by Neurosyphilis

Symptom: dementia with progressive cognitive impairment

Descriptive Diagnosis: dementia

Actual Diagnosis: neurosyphilis

Stealth Infection: *Treponema pallidum*

Tests to Consider: blood tests or spinal fluid tests for syphilis

Potential Treatment: antibiotics

Case in Point: It is generally recommended that persons who develop symptoms of dementia have certain blood tests to rule out treatable causes of dementia. One of these is a blood test for syphilis. Though rarely found these days, on occasion a person will have a long-standing syphilis infection that they were not aware of, which is the cause of their gradually evolving dementia.

Dementia and Other Neurological Problems, Accompanied by Diarrhea and Weight Loss Due to Whipple's Disease

Symptom: progressive memory loss, confusion, balance problems, and weight loss, diarrhea

Descriptive Diagnosis: dementia

Actual Diagnosis: Whipple's disease

Stealth Infection: *Tropheryma whippelii*

Tests to Consider: small bowel biopsy

Potential Treatment: antibiotics

Case in Point: A rare person who is developing dementia has had ongoing gastrointestinal symptoms and some weight loss. Often these symptoms are attributed to the dementia. Also, some of the currently used medicines for treating Alzheimer's disease can cause diarrhea and weight loss. However, if diarrhea and weight loss predated the onset of the memory and brain problems or the use of anti-dementia medicines, Whipple's disease should be considered.

Schizophrenia Linked to Exposure to Certain Infections Such as Toxoplasmosis

Symptom: neuropsychiatric symptoms including disordered thinking, delusions, and hallucinations, starting in young adulthood and remaining chronic and disabling

Descriptive Diagnosis: schizophrenia

Actual Diagnosis: schizophrenia triggered by infectious exposure

Stealth Infection: *Toxoplasma gondii*

Tests to Consider: blood tests available

Potential Treatment: antibiotics

Case in Point: Persons with recent-onset schizophrenia often show evidence of exposure to *Toxoplasma gondii*. Also, mothers of schizophrenic patients show increased likelihood of exposure to this organism. Toxoplasma infection can sometimes lead to psychotic symptoms similar to schizophrenia. It is estimated that up to one third of the world's population has had exposure to toxoplasma infection. Even if evidence of exposure to the infection is found, treatment of a person with established schizophrenia for toxoplasma infection likely will not help. Toxoplasma dormant in the system can suddenly flare up or emerge in persons with significant immune deficiencies such as AIDS.

Schizophrenia and Infection with Herpesvirus

Symptom: neuropsychiatric symptoms including disordered thinking, delusions, and hallucinations, starting in young adulthood, and remaining chronic and disabling

Descriptive Diagnosis: schizophrenia

Actual Diagnosis: infectious encephalopathy causing schizophrenia

Stealth Infection: human endogenous retrovirus (HERV-W) and herpes simplex virus type 2, or cytomegalovirus

Tests to Consider: blood or serum tests for the viruses

Potential Treatment: antiherpesvirus medicine valacyclovir may reduce the symptoms of some individuals with schizophrenia

Case in Point: Persons with recent onset of schizophrenia often show some evidence of exposure to these organisms. Also, mothers of schizophrenic patients show increased likelihood of exposure to these organisms. In the future, those with schizophrenia and their families will likely have an evaluation with attention to infections they carry.

Herpesvirus Spreading to the Brain

Symptom: rapidly progressive encephalitis with confusion, delirium, seizures, without exposure to others with meningitis or encephalitis

Descriptive Diagnosis: encephalitis, seizures

Actual Diagnosis: herpes encephalitis

Stealth Infection: herpes simplex virus

Tests to Consider: spinal fluid examination for the virus

Potential Treatment: antiviral medicines used to treat herpesvirus

Case in Point: A person may develop rapid-onset confusion, difficulty walking, seizures, and other severe neurological symptoms without history of outside exposure. They may or may not have a significant recent history of cold sores or herpesvirus infections. However, herpesvirus carried in one's own system may suddenly spread to the brain. Herpes encephalitis can leave persons with permanent brain damage.

Lyme Disease Causes Neurological Problems

Symptom: difficulty thinking, brain fatigue

Descriptive Diagnosis: cognitive impairment, chronic fatigue, depression

Actual Diagnosis: Lyme disease

Stealth Infection: *Borrelia burgdorferi*

Tests to Consider: serum tests for Lyme disease

Potential Treatment: antibiotics for Lyme disease

Case in Point: Persons with untreated Lyme disease may experience a wide range of neurological symptoms, including changes in mood, memory loss, sleep disturbance, and brain fatigue. There may be dizziness, wooziness, tingling and other sensory disturbances, muscle twitching, and symptoms of neuropathy. Many of these symptoms are attributed to various other causes until the diagnosis is correctly made.

Brain problems caused by AIDS

Symptom: confusion, difficulty thinking

Descriptive Diagnosis: encephalopathy, dementia, delirium

Actual Diagnosis: AIDS encephalopathy

Stealth Infection: human immunodeficiency virus (HIV)

Tests to Consider: HIV test, spinal fluid test

Potential Treatment: antiviral medications used for AIDS

Case in Point: AIDS is known to cause major neurological problems, including confusion, often accompanied by some problems with balance and coordination and altered behavior. The effect of this virus on the brain is often compounded by coexisting infections such as herpes, toxoplasmosis, or other organisms that the person may carry.

Epilepsy Linked to Tropical Infections

Symptom: grand mal seizure (epilepsy)

Descriptive Diagnosis: epilepsy

Actual Diagnosis: infectious encephalopathy with seizures

Stealth Infection: *Plasmodium falciparum*, helminthic infection, cysticercosis, others

Tests to Consider: various specific tests for these organisms

Potential Treatment: various anti-infectives

Case in Point: Persons living in tropical countries, especially in rural and medically underserved areas of these countries, may be exposed to a variety of infections, including parasitic infections and malaria. For someone who has resided in such an area, new-onset seizure disorder is often the result of infection with one of many such organisms. The presence of these infections should be sought in consultation with an infectious disease specialist.

Rapidly Progressive Dementia Due to Contagious Prion in Creutzfeldt-Jakob Disease

Symptom: rapidly progressive memory loss and confusion

Descriptive Diagnosis: dementia, progressive multifocal leukoencephalopathy

Actual Diagnosis: Creutzfeldt–Jakob disease

Stealth Infection: transmissible prion

Tests to Consider: cerebrospinal fluid examination, electroencephalogram

Potential Treatment: none

Case in Point: A transmissible prion particle has been identified as the cause of Creutzfeldt-Jakob disease. Prions also cause the lesser-known Gerstmann-Sträussler-Scheinker syndrome, kuru, fatal familial insomnia, as well as animal diseases such as bovine spongiform encephalopathy (mad cow disease), and chronic wasting disease in elk. On very rare occasion, such conditions have been transmitted by transplantation of infected tissues such as corneal graft in the case of Creutzfeldt-Jakob disease.

Lymphocytic Choriomeningitis Virus Infection Related to Organ Transplantation

Symptom: most often no symptoms; otherwise encephalitis, meningitis

Descriptive Diagnosis: encephalitis, meningitis

Actual Diagnosis: viral encephalopathy

Stealth Infection: Lymphocytic Choriomeningitis Virus (LCMV)

Tests to Consider: none commonly available

Potential Treatment: none

Case in Point: In May 2005 the deaths of several organ transplant patients in the U.S. were linked to this virus. The virus is carried by rodents, including mice and hamsters, and normally has little effect on healthy persons. However, in those whose immune system is suppressed, it can cause very significant illness.

Breast Disease

Now that cancer of the female cervix has been linked to a virus, other female cancers are also being scrutinized for infectious triggers. Breast cancer is one of those cancers. Though evidence is preliminary, an infectious source is being considered as one potential cause or contributing factor in some cases.

Breast Cancer in Some Cases Linked to Mammary Tumor Virus

Symptom: breast cancer

Descriptive Diagnosis: breast cancer

Actual Diagnosis: breast cancer triggered by virus

Stealth Infection: human mammary tumor virus

Tests to Consider: none routinely available

Potential Treatment: none for the virus; conventional treatment of the breast cancer

Case in Point: Mouse mammary tumor virus (MMTV) causes breast cancer in mice. The human mammary tumor virus (HMTV) is 95 percent genetically identical to the MMTV. There is indication that up to one third of women with breast cancer have a gene segment in their breast tissue corresponding to this virus. Moreover, more than two thirds of tumor samples from women with a particular type of breast cancer, called inflammatory breast cancer, have similar evidence of this virus. This virus-disease association is far from proven, but is an active area of investigation.

Cancers Linked to Stealth Infections

A very important recent advance in medicine is the emerging evidence of the relationship between certain infections and cancer. This possibility was raised a hundred years ago. However, because it is generally not possible to obtain direct proof using Koch's postulates, the cause-and-effect relationship has been viewed with skepticism. Modern methods and cumulative evidence are providing convincing results for such an association in several types of cancer.

An important implication of these findings is that vaccines against the germs that are involved could reduce the likelihood of developing various cancers. A vaccine against the human papillomavirus, the virus that can cause cancer of the female cervix, is currently available. The concept and practice of using vaccinations to prevent cancers may be one of the significant accomplishments of twenty-first-century medicine.

Cancer of the Cervix in Women Caused by Human Papillomavirus

Symptom: none; finding of an abnormal Pap smear test

Descriptive Diagnosis: cancer of the cervix

Actual Diagnosis: cancer of cervix due to virus infection

Stealth Infection: human papillomavirus (HPV)

Tests to Consider: annual Pap smear tests, biopsy, tests for the virus

Potential Treatment: conventional treatment for cancer of the cervix; topical treatments are available for venereal warts; vaccination to prevent the viral infection is available

Case in Point: Most cancers of the cervix evolve from pelvic infection with the human papillomavirus, usually acquired through sexual relations. Venereal warts may or may not be visible. Sometimes the first indication that something is wrong is the finding of "atypical cells of undetermined significance" (ASCUS) on a Pap smear test. Women with such findings should be carefully checked for pelvic infections, and if an infection is found, prompt treatment and protection against possible reinfection from a partner who may harbor infectious organisms are warranted.

Cancer of the Liver Caused by Hepatitis Virus(es)

Symptom: none for many years, followed by symptoms of liver cancer

Descriptive Diagnosis: cancer of the liver

Actual Diagnosis: cancer of the liver triggered by virus

Stealth Infection: hepatitis B virus, hepatitis C virus

Tests to Consider: hepatitis B and hepatitis C blood tests, tests for liver cancer in persons with long-standing chronic infection with these viruses

Potential Treatment: conventional treatment for liver cancer; immunotherapy and antiviral therapy may be considered for persistent infection with the viruses before cancer develops; a vaccine against hepatitis B is available

Case in Point: Hepatitis B is endemic to Southeast Asia and some other parts of the world. Both hepatitis B and hepatitis C are commonly found in asymptomatic persons who may or may not have slight elevation of their blood test which checks the liver chemistries. Persons with long-standing infection with these viruses have significantly increased likelihood of developing cancer of the liver.

Cancer of the Lymph Nodes, Lymphoma Caused by Mononucleosis Virus

Symptom: usual symptoms of lymphoma in persons who may or may not have had a history of mononucleosis

Descriptive Diagnosis: Burkitt's lymphoma, Hodgkin's lymphoma, non-Hodgkin's lymphoma, nasopharyngeal carcinoma

Actual Diagnosis: lymphoma due to virus infection

Stealth Infection: Epstein-Barr virus (member of the herpesvirus family)

Tests to Consider: biopsy of the lymph nodes and serum tests for the virus

Potential Treatment: treatment available for the cancers; early cases of mononucleosis have been reported to respond partly to antiviral medicine

Case in Point: The mononucleosis virus (Epstein-Barr virus) has been linked to several cancers. So-called Burkitt's lymphoma was the first to be linked to this virus. This cancer is especially likely in persons living in Africa or tropical countries who are also infected with malaria. This virus has been linked to many other human cancers including hematopoietic, epithelial, and mesenchymal tumors.

Sarcoma, a Rare Form of Cancer Caused by Herpesvirus in Immunosuppressed Individuals

Symptom: usual symptoms of Kaposi's sarcoma (rapidly growing and spreading colored nodules under the skin and mucous membranes such as the mouth)

Descriptive Diagnosis: Kaposi's sarcoma

Actual Diagnosis: Kaposi's sarcoma due to herpesvirus

Stealth Infection: human herpesvirus type 8

Tests to Consider: biopsy

Potential Treatment: treatment available for sarcoma; antivirals available against herpesviruses

Case in Point: Persons who have AIDS or patients who are immuno-suppressed should be careful to avoid herpesvirus exposure, and should receive treatment for herpesvirus infections when they are present. Herpesvirus 8 in such individuals is the cause of this highly dangerous form of cancer.

Stomach Cancer Linked to Ulcer Bacteria

Symptom: many years of chronic acid indigestion, followed by symptoms of stomach cancer

Descriptive Diagnosis: stomach cancer

Actual Diagnosis: stomach cancer triggered by *H. pylori*

Stealth Infection: *Helicobacter pylori*

Tests to Consider: usual tests for *H. pylori* and stomach cancer

Potential Treatment: treatment available for stomach cancer; early treatment of *H. pylori* with antibiotics

Case in Point: One reason to treat persons who have *H. pylori* is because of the strong suspicion that long-term infection of the stomach with *H. pylori* predisposes the patient to cancer of the stomach. Decline in the incidence of stomach cancer in recent years has been attributed to the treatment and eradication of *H. pylori* from carriers of this stealth germ.

Leukemia and Lymphoma Caused by Viruses

Symptom: none for many years, then usual symptoms and findings of leukemia or lymphoma

Descriptive Diagnosis: adult T-cell leukemia or lymphoma

Actual Diagnosis: leukemia or lymphoma triggered by viruses

Stealth Infection: human T-cell lymphotropic virus type I (HTLV-I)

Tests to Consider: test for the virus is available, but not commonly done

Potential Treatment: treatment is available for the cancers; no specific antiviral medicine is currently available for the virus

Case in Point: Viruses are increasingly investigated as agents that contribute to the development of cancers of the blood and lymphatic system. HTLV-I is a prime candidate in adult T-cell leukemia. Furthermore, *H. pylori* has been implicated in cases of B-cell lymphoma. *Borrelia burgdorferi* causing Lyme disease is also suspected to be a factor in cutaneous B-cell lymphoma.

Hodgkin's Disease Linked to Cytomegalovirus

Symptom: fever and lymph node enlargement

Descriptive Diagnosis: Hodgkin's disease

Actual Diagnosis: Hodgkin's disease associated with cytomegalovirus

Stealth Infection: cytomegalovirus (CMV), a member of the herpesvirus family

Tests to Consider: serum tests for cytomegalovirus

Potential Treatment: antiviral medicine specific for CMV available

Case in Point: A patient who was very healthy all of his life until his late eighties, received a blood transfusion after a surgical procedure. Some time later, he developed night sweats. His CT scan showed enlarged lymph nodes, which were biopsied, and he was diagnosed with Hodgkin's disease. He was started on chemotherapy. Soon afterward, he developed severe cytomegalovirus pneumonia. Current investigations are pursuing the possibility that the Epstein-Barr virus and possibly cytomegalovirus might play a role in the development of some cases of Hodgkin's disease. Both Epstein-Barr and cytomegalovirus are members of the herpesvirus family.

Cholangiocarcinoma Caused by Liver Flukes

Symptom: long-standing symptoms of parasitic liver flukes (worms) in tropical countries, followed by the usual symptoms of cancer of the bile ducts

Descriptive Diagnosis: cholangiocarcinoma, or cancer of the biliary system

Actual Diagnosis: cholangiocarcinoma caused by liver flukes

Stealth Infection: *Opisthorchis viverrini* and *Clonorchis sinensis* (liver flukes)

Tests to Consider: usual tests for parasites, including stool tests for the ova

Potential Treatment: treatment for the cancer is available, as well as treatment for the liver parasites

Case in Point: Cholangiocarcinoma is a rare cancer of the bile ducts in the biliary system. Liver fluke–associated cholangiocarcinoma is a significant problem in developing countries. Infestation with liver flukes is rare in nonrural areas of industrialized countries, however.

Squamous Cancer of the Bladder Linked to Parasitic Infection

Symptom: none, or blood in the urine

Descriptive Diagnosis: bladder cancer

Actual Diagnosis: bladder cancer caused by parasitic infection

Stealth Infection: *Schistosoma haematobium*

Tests to Consider: urine test for the parasite

Potential Treatment: usual treatment for the bladder cancer; medicines available to treat the parasite

Case in Point: Long-standing infection with various infectious organisms predisposes to cancer. Schistosomiasis invades the bladder, and eventually causes cancer of the bladder if left untreated. This infection is found commonly in rural areas of tropical countries.

Ear Conditions

Stealth infections are rarely found in the ear, although viruses may be involved in some cases of sudden hearing loss or vertigo. Some skin conditions of the ear canal are outlined below, because these skin infections are not always properly identified and treated.

Sudden Hearing Loss May be Due to Stealth Viruses

Symptom: sudden loss of hearing in one ear without any accompanying symptoms

Descriptive Diagnosis: acute hearing loss of unknown cause

Actual Diagnosis: injury to the hearing nerve triggered by virus

Stealth Infection: herpesviruses including cytomegalovirus

Tests to Consider: blood tests for the viruses

Potential Treatment: antiviral medicines against herpesvirus are available; other treatments for acute hearing loss may also be given in the form of a short course of corticosteroids

Case in Point: Most of the time sudden hearing loss is labeled "idiopathic," meaning due to no identifiable cause, because is it is not possible to get a sample from the nerve to see what may be affecting it. However, there is suspicion that herpesviruses may be involved. Various herpesviruses have also been implicated in other nerve palsies, such as Bell's palsy and Ramsay Hunt syndrome. Members of the herpesvirus family that may be involved include herpes simplex, *Herpes zoster*, cytomegalovirus, as well as Epstein-Barr virus.

Vertigo due to Viral Labyrinthitis

Symptom: sudden-onset vertigo (dizziness with a spinning feeling)

Descriptive Diagnosis: acute labyrinthitis, vertigo

Actual Diagnosis: labyrinthitis due to virus infection

Stealth Infection: herpesviruses (and others, such as mumps, rubella)

Tests to Consider: blood tests for herpesviruses

Potential Treatment: antiviral medicine against herpesvirus is available; treatment and management for vertigo is available

Case in Point: Most cases of vertigo, a medical term meaning spinning dizziness, affecting adults are due to an otolith (floater) in the inner ear, which becomes entangled in the sensors in the inner ear, causing a feeling of spinning dizziness. However, in young children, vertigo may be the result of viral labyrinthitis caused by herpesviruses, cytomegalovirus, Epstein-Barr virus, mumps, rubella, or others. If you have cold sores, genital herpes, or had exposure to cytomegalovirus, and develop vertigo, brief treatment with an anti-herpes antiviral medication may be considered.

Dandruff of the Ear Canal

Symptom: itchy, flaky skin in the ear canals

Descriptive Diagnosis: dry skin, otitis externa

Actual Diagnosis: seborrheic dermatitis

Stealth Infection: Malassezia ovale

Tests to Consider: none

Potential Treatment: antifungal preparation

Case in Point: In adults the skin of the ear canal often becomes dry and scaly. Often this is due to water and soap that gets in the ear as we shower or bathe, and is not washed and dried in the same way as the rest of the skin. However, those with dandruff (due to seborrheic dermatitis) of the scalp, eyebrows, or cheeks can also develop similar seborrheic dermatitis in the skin of the ear canal. One remedy is to treat the *Malassezia ovale*, which is the fungus believed to play a significant role in perpetuating seborrheic dermatitis.

Swimmer's Ear Nonresponsive to Antibacterial Eardrops

Symptom: persistent swimmer's ear, not improved with antibacterial eardrops

Descriptive Diagnosis: swimmer's ear attributed to bacteria such as pseudomonas or staphylococcus

Actual Diagnosis: fungal infection of the ear canal

Stealth Infection: aspergillus, actinomyces, yeast

Tests to Consider: examination and culture of the material in the ear canal

Potential Treatment: treatment with appropriate antifungal medication

Case in Point: Persons who enjoy spending time in the water are familiar with "swimmer's ear," an irritation of the skin of the ear canal from water that pools in the ear canal for extended periods of time. On occasion, the irritation of the ear canal becomes persistent and more severe. When consulted, most doctors treat the problem with antibacterial remedies. However, if the condition does not respond to the usual therapy, then certain fungal colonies or yeast may be the culprit, rather than bacteria. Specific antifungal treatment may be the proper remedy.

Endocrine System

Endocrine problems used to be called glandular problems, and include conditions such as diabetes, thyroid disease, conditions of the adrenal glands, and hormonal conditions. Active ongoing stealth infections generally do not affect the endocrine system. However, there is increasing evidence that certain viral infections may act in a hit-and-run fashion to trigger the immune system to attack one's own endocrine organs.

Such a mechanism is believed to play a role in the development of conditions such as juvenile (Type 1) diabetes, and inflammation of the thyroid (thyroiditis), which may lead to both overactive, and eventually underactive thyroid conditions. Rarely, tuberculosis can affect the adrenal glands.

Virus May Trigger Childhood Diabetes

Symptom: typical symptoms of juvenile-onset diabetes

Descriptive Diagnosis: Type 1 diabetes

Actual Diagnosis: Type 1 diabetes possibly triggered by virus

Stealth Infection: Coxsackie B enterovirus, congenital rubella virus, mumps (all suspected)

Tests to Consider: serology tests are available, but may not be helpful

Potential Treatment: none for the viruses; usual treatment for diabetes

Case in Point: Coxsackie B enterovirus is implicated in triggering the immune response that attacks the beta cells of the pancreas, causing juvenile-onset diabetes. Enteroviruses infect 50 million people in the U.S. annually. Other viruses that are potential triggers for type 1 diabetes are mumps and congenital rubella virus. At this time there is no treatment for these viruses. In research settings, attempts have been made to modify the body's immune response to the viral trigger to mitigate the resultant damage to the beta cells of the pancreas, which normally produce the body's insulin.

Inflammation of the Thyroid (Thyroiditis) and Viruses

Symptom: usual symptoms of overactive thyroid, such as shakiness, palpitations, weight loss

Descriptive Diagnosis: subacute thyroiditis

Actual Diagnosis: subacute thyroiditis possibly triggered by virus infection

Stealth Infection: mumps virus, influenza virus, hepatitis C virus, or respiratory viruses (suspected)

Tests to Consider: serology tests available, though not helpful

Potential Treatment: none, except for acute influenza; antiviral treatment for other infections is not available currently

Case in Point: Thyroiditis may be due to an inflammatory reaction triggered by viruses. It appears to be an autoimmune process, whereby the body causes an excessive inflammatory response within the thyroid gland in response to a viral infection. In this process, the thyroid becomes inflamed and excessive amounts of thyroid hormone leak into the blood, causing symptoms of hyperthyroidism. After a while this process subsides, and when the injured thyroid gland is unable to manufacture sufficient amounts of thyroid hormone, an underactive thyroid condition, or hypothyroidism, may result. The offending viruses appear to act in a hit-and-run fashion, triggering an immune reaction, then disappearing from the body, and not remaining as a lingering infection.

Adrenal Insufficiency (Addison's Disease) Due to Tuberculosis as a Rare Cause

Symptom: usual symptoms and findings of adrenal insufficiency in someone who may not recall prior tuberculosis infection or exposure

Descriptive Diagnosis: adrenal insufficiency of unknown cause

Actual Diagnosis: adrenal insufficiency due to damage to the adrenal glands by tuberculous infection

Stealth Infection: *Mycobacterium tuberculosis*

Tests to Consider: TB skin test, chest X-ray, CT of adrenal glands

Potential Treatment: treatment of adrenal insufficiency is available; tuberculosis infection can be treated with antituberculous antimicrobials

Case in Point: Persons infected with tuberculosis or exposed to TB sometimes develop a localized infection in the adrenal gland caused by the tuberculosis microorganism. The infection of the gland can injure the gland, resulting in adrenal insufficiency, known as Addison's disease. Adrenal insufficiency is most often caused by processes other than tuberculosis. Tubercular cause of the condition is more commonly seen in areas of the world where tuberculosis infections are widespread. In patients with AIDS, cytomegalovirus infection accounts for more than 50 percent of cases of adrenal insufficiency. Other pathogens that can cause adrenal insufficiency in patients with AIDS include *Mycobacterium avium-intracellulare*, fungi, toxoplasma organisms, and *Pneumocystis* organisms.

Esophagus

See also section on Mouth and Throat.

Stealth infections of the esophagus in otherwise healthy individuals are uncommon. However, a couple of conditions that may be overlooked are yeast colonization in persons with other medical conditions or who are on medications that predispose to yeast infections. There is also the possibility of recurrent cold sores in the esophagus due to herpesvirus. Many noninfectious conditions such as canker sores (Behcet's disease) or acid reflux can also cause problems and symptoms in the esophagus.

Yeast Colonization of the Esophagus in Diabetics or Those on Corticosteroids

Symptom: persistent heartburn and burning in the esophagus that has not been responsive to antacids in a person with diabetes or on corticosteroids or on antibiotics

Descriptive Diagnosis: GERD, esophagitis, heartburn

Actual Diagnosis: yeast infection of the esophagus (candida esophagitis)

Stealth Infection: *Candida albicans*

Tests to Consider: endoscopic examination of esophagus

Potential Treatment: antiyeast preparations; consider empiric treatment

Case in Point: A typical case may be a patient with asthma who has had a series of severe respiratory infections. Antibiotics along with prednisone were given over a few weeks. The patient had a history of acid indigestion and acid reflux. However, as he continues to take his medications, the acid indigestion becomes progressively worse. Antacids do not seem to work, and the patient suffers terribly from the pain in the esophagus, which is blamed on the irritant effect from the prednisone and the antibiotics. He is told to continue antacids. Finally yeast overgrowth of the esophagus is considered and empiric treatment with anti-fungal medicine given in the suspension form promptly relieves the symptoms.

Episodic Burning in the Esophagus and Pain on Swallowing

Symptom: episodes of burning pain in the upper esophagus or throat on swallowing that last a few days, and which soon go away but reappear weeks or months later

Descriptive Diagnosis: esophagitis, GERD, globus hystericus

Actual Diagnosis: recurrent cold sores

Stealth Infection: herpes simplex

Tests to Consider: endoscopy and viral culture at the time of symptoms

Potential Treatment: antiviral given for herpes infections

Case in Point: A person may have episodes of quite unpleasant pain way in the back of the throat or in the upper esophagus where it hurts to swallow. It feels like the sore area is localized to a well-defined spot, rather than the entire esophagus. After a few days the pain disappears, only to recur again a few weeks or few months later. Persons who were exposed to the herpesvirus may in fact have the cold sores in the esophagus, and not around the mouth. Canker sores may also appear in the esophagus and cause similar symptoms.

Bad Breath, Pain on Swallowing in the Upper Esophagus in Older Persons

Symptom: recurrent bad breath (halitosis) and pain in the upper esophagus when swallowing; occasionally a pill or some food swallowed earlier reappears in the back of the throat

Descriptive Diagnosis: bad breath due to mouth bacteria, spasms of the esophagus, GERD

Actual Diagnosis: infected Zenker's diverticulum

Stealth Infection: mouth bacteria

Tests to Consider: X-ray of esophagus

Potential Treatment: antibiotics or surgery may be needed

Case in Point: This condition is present in a few older persons. In addition to the bad breath, which is often blamed on the condition of the teeth and gums, pills or foodstuffs that are swallowed may reappear in the throat after a delayed period. At times, discomfort with swallowing is noted. Eventually an esophagram (or "swallowing X-ray") is done, which shows a small pouch called a Zenker's diverticulum (see Glossary) in the upper esophagus. Festering foodstuffs or saliva residue in this abnormal pouch in the esophagus is partially responsible for the bad breath.

Eye

The eyeball is rarely a target of stealth infections. However, certain conditions that may emerge out of hiding and infect the eyes, including shingles (*Herpes zoster*) and toxoplasmosis are described below. A condition called blepharitis of the eyelids and eyelashes may be caused by conditions treatable with antibiotics.

Chronically Irritated Eyelids Due to Rosacea

Symptom: persistent irritation of the eyelashes, dry eye syndrome, plugging of the tear ducts

Descriptive Diagnosis: chronic blepharitis, plugged tear ducts

Actual Diagnosis: rosacea affecting the eye

Stealth Infection: no infectious organism proven, but rosacea responds to antibiotic treatment

Tests to Consider: no tests; observed by examination

Potential Treatment: antibiotics

Case in Point: A 90-year-old patient was diagnosed with chronic

blepharitis, as well as dry eye syndrome. No specific cause was identified. However, her physician considered the possibility of rosacea
blepharitis. The patient was treated with doxycycline for three
months. During and after this treatment, there was significant
improvement of her eye symptoms, though not a complete cure.
Rosacea is not caused by a known infection, nor is it believed to be
contagious. Nevertheless, it responds to antibiotics including doxycycline and metronidazole. Untreated rosacea blepharitis can cause
plugging of the tear ducts, causing overflow of tears, or can damage
the tear glands and cause dry eye syndrome in older persons. Left
untreated, severe cases may impair the vision.

Rapidly Progressive Inflammation in the Eye Due to Reemergent Toxoplasmosis

Symptom: progressive inflammation of the eye causing vision loss in
person treated with immunosuppressants

Descriptive Diagnosis: endophthalmitis, retinitis, uveitis

Actual Diagnosis: toxoplasmosis of the eye

Stealth Infection: *Toxoplasma gondii*

Tests to Consider: blood test, culture of fluid from the eye

Potential Treatment: specific antimicrobial available

Case in Point: An elderly man who was treated with prednisone for
an unrelated condition developed a painful inflammation within his
eyeball, which caused rapid deterioration of his vision. His symptoms
did not respond to anti-inflammatories. He was diagnosed by his
eye doctor with chorioretinitis, most likely caused by an infection,
and a small sample of fluid from his eye was taken. Toxoplasmosis
infection was confirmed. Toxoplasmosis exposure is common in the
general population, but rarely causes symptoms in healthy individuals. However, sudden emergence of the organism in the form of

potentially devastating toxoplasma infections in the eyes or brain can occur in patients who are on immunosuppressant medicines, or in those with immune deficiencies such as AIDS.

Pain in the Eye Followed by Appearance of Blisters Due to Shingles

Symptom: pain around the eye, followed days later by painful blistery eruption around the eye and partly in the eye

Descriptive Diagnosis: shingles

Actual Diagnosis: herpes zoster ophthalmicus

Stealth Infection: *Varicella zoster* virus

Tests to Consider: not usually necessary; fluid from blisters can be tested for the virus

Potential Treatment: antiviral against herpesviruses

Case in Point: A shingles eruption in and around the eye requires very prompt treatment to avoid injury to the eye and the vision. Diagnosis and treatment are sometimes delayed because pain around the eye, which develops a few days before the rash erupts, is misattributed to other causes. Treatment is usually under the care of an eye specialist. A vaccine is available that is effective in preventing shingles.

Dandruff of the Eyebrows and Eyelashes Linked to Fungus

Symptom: dandruff of the eyebrows and eyelashes

Descriptive Diagnosis: seborrheic blepharitis

Actual Diagnosis: seborrheic blepharitis in part due to fungal colonization

Stealth Infection: *Malassezia ovale* (suspected)

Tests to Consider: no testing is used

Potential Treatment: antifungal shampoo, cream, medication

Case in Point: The skin of the scalp, chest, and ears, as well as the eyebrows and eyelids can be affected by seborrheic dermatitis, related to a fungal infection. In addition to the usual creams and lotions soothing to the skin, specific antifungal treatment for this condition may be helpful.

Fatigue and Malaise

See also section on Blood and Lymphatic diseases.

Feeling poorly is a symptom common to most chronic medical conditions. Most of us hope that if we don't feel well, a treatable cause can be identified and remedied. In numerous cases, such a pathologic cause cannot be clearly established. In such cases, certain labels are assigned for purposes of classification. Chronic fatigue syndrome (CFS) and Gulf War syndrome are puzzling conditions where efforts have been focused to find possible underlying stealth infections. It has been suggested that chronic fatigue syndrome may be a post-infectious condition, as it sometimes starts and evolves rapidly after an influenzalike onset, especially during the winter months. Even so, persistence of known infectious agents in persons with CFS has not been shown. Fibromyalgia is another condition that has not yet been attributed to a clear-cut cause. However, there are infectious conditions such as Lyme disease that produce symptoms similar to CFS. Other stealth infections that may cause persistent or recurrent malaise are discussed below.

Cytomegalovirus Causing Relapsing Fatigue

Symptom: chronic recurrent fatigue

Descriptive Diagnosis: chronic fatigue syndrome, fibromyalgia

Actual Diagnosis: chronic relapsing cytomegalovirus infection

Stealth Infection: cytomegalovirus (suspected)

Tests to Consider: blood tests or urine test for cytomegalovirus

Potential Treatment: antiviral medicines (used against herpesviruses)

Case in Point: A patient who had complained of persistent recurrent fatigue saw her doctor. Most of her laboratory tests were normal, but blood titers for cytomegalovirus IgG and IgM were elevated, showing evidence of exposure to the virus. She was prescribed valacyclovir, an antiviral used mostly to treat other herpesviruses that has activity against cytomegalovirus, also known as human herpesvirus 5. Very soon after starting the medicine she felt significantly improved and most of her energy returned. The syndrome of frailty in geriatric patients has been linked to chronic cytomegalovirus infection.

Syphilis Can Cause Malaise and Lead to Long-term Medical Problems

Symptom: fatigue, malaise, transient skin rash, memory problems

Descriptive Diagnosis: chronic fatigue, dementia

Actual Diagnosis: syphilis

Stealth Infection: *Treponema pallidum*

Tests to Consider: usual blood tests or spinal fluid tests for syphilis

Potential Treatment: antibiotics

Case in Point: Syphilis is the "great masquerader." Those who carry it in their system may have long-standing nonspecific symptoms. Syphilis was discussed in more detail in the section on Brain and Psychiatric Conditions.

Lyme Disease Causing Chronic Fatigue

Symptom: fatigue and nervous system symptoms such as mental fatigue, headaches, or memory problems

Descriptive Diagnosis: chronic fatigue syndrome, fibromyalgia

Actual Diagnosis: Lyme disease

Stealth Infection: *Borrelia burgdorferi*

Tests to Consider: antibody or other tests specific for Lyme disease

Potential Treatment: antibiotics specific for Lyme disease

Case in Point: The initial symptom is a patchy skin rash (erythema chronicum migrans), which soon disappears without treatment. The rash is followed within several days or weeks by recurrent, scattered joint pains. After that, the chronic fatigue and achiness may be the predominant symptom, and the other symptoms fade in memory. The patient is often diagnosed to have fibromyalgia or chronic fatigue syndrome. Antibiotics, though available, may not always be helpful if started too late.

Hepatitis B or C Causing Fatigue

Symptom: mild generalized fatigue or malaise

Descriptive Diagnosis: chronic fatigue syndrome, fibromyalgia

Actual Diagnosis: chronic hepatitis B or C infection

Stealth Infection: hepatitis B or C

Tests to Consider: blood tests for chronic hepatitis

Potential Treatment: treatment available with immunotherapy

Case in Point: After exposure, the only symptom of carrying these viruses may be minor—mostly a feeling that one doesn't feel quite as well and energetic as one used to. Other times, there may be fatigue, some weight loss, and muscle pains, in which case the ailment is often labeled fibromyalgia. In some cases, chronic hepatitis C carrier state can lead to more severe problems, including thyroiditis, vasculitis, kidney disease such as glomerulonephritis, inflammatory rheumatism, thrombocytopenia, and lymphomalike conditions.

Chronic Fatigue Syndrome Attributed in Some to Mycoplasma or Chlamydia

Symptom: fatigue, malaise, achiness

Descriptive Diagnosis: chronic fatigue syndrome, fibromyalgia

Actual Diagnosis: chronic chlamydia or mycoplasma infection

Stealth Infection: mycoplasma or chlamydia (suspected)

Tests to Consider: serology blood test

Potential Treatment: antibiotics

Case in Point: Mycoplasma titers are elevated in some people with chronic fatigue. This does not necessarily prove active infection, only that they had prior exposure to the organism. One patient had a long history of fibromyalgia. This developed after she had an episode of what was diagnosed as viral pleurisy, because routine bacterial cultures of the pleural fluid were reported to be negative. The pleurisy resolved, but she never felt well afterwards. A year later the "viral pleurisy" returned. The pleurisy fluid was drained, and the lung symptoms resolved. However, she continued to have fatigue, malaise, and achiness, which she did not have prior to the original episode. Eventually various specific serology tests were done to look for exposure to organisms that can cause pleurisy. Based on elevated mycoplasma and chlamydia titers, the antibiotic doxycycline was given empirically. Her decade-long fibromyalgia syndrome resolved.

Feet and Ankles

See also sections on Stealth Infections and the Skin, and Arthritis and Joints.
Older persons often develop rusty-colored discoloration of the skin

around their feet and ankles. The name of this condition is stasis dermatitis. It is not caused by infection. However, infections can overrun the abnormal skin. Cellulitis, a condition caused by skin bacteria infecting areas of broken skin, can be caused by an opportunistic bacterial infection entering the skin damaged by the stasis dermatitis. Fungal infections, such as *Tinea pedis* (athlete's foot) can also overrun the abnormal skin.

Often, bacterial and fungal infections can be present simultaneously as an example of dual infection. One of these conditions is usually diagnosed, but the other might be hidden in plain sight and overlooked. When both infections are present, both need to be treated in order to cure the problem.

Rust-colored Skin and Poorly Healing Sores Around the Ankles Compounded by Skin Fungus

Symptom: dry, leathery, rust-colored skin around the ankles, with poorly healing sores

Descriptive Diagnosis: stasis dermatitis, cellulitis, lipodermatosclerosis

Actual Diagnosis: tinea colonization of the abnormal skin in addition to stasis dermatitis

Stealth Infection: *Tinea corporis*

Tests to Consider: fungal culture of skin

Potential Treatment: antifungal creams or pills

Case in Point: This condition usually happens in older persons, or in those with chronically swollen ankles. The skin around the ankles becomes dry and develops a rust-colored appearance, and may become hardened and leathery (the name of this advanced stage of the skin condition is lipodermatosclerosis). If the skin is injured, an open skin sore will form. If the open sore heals poorly and persists, it is usually treated with skin ulcer care. If bacterial infection is suspected, antibacterials are used.

In addition, the skin in the area may also show signs of athlete's foot fungus, and the toenails may show signs of onychomycosis, or nail fungus. The skin affected by the athlete's foot fungus often extends into the area of stasis dermatitis. Yet most of the attention is focused on bacteria, and treatment of the fungal infection is often neglected. Treatment of both conditions has to be undertaken at the same time, along with meticulous skin and wound care, in order for the skin sore to heal.

Gynecologic and Pelvic Conditions
See also section on Urinary Tract and Bladder Conditions.
Stealth germs may go undetected and untreated for extended periods in the female pelvic area because of vague and nonspecific symptoms, which may resemble menstrual cramps or discomfort. Vaginal discharge may be minimal, or there may be no symptoms at all. Yet undetected and untreated infections can cause problems, including infertility, infections to a developing fetus, or to the newborn during birth. After extended periods of time cancer can develop, such as cancer of the cervix caused by the human papillomavirus. Even if treated, sexually transmitted infections may be repeatedly reacquired from a partner who also harbors these organisms, but may be an asymptomatic carrier.

It has been pointed out by thoughtful diagnosticians that pelvic inflammatory disease is easy to miss. It is sometimes confused with other gynecological disorders. No single test can detect all cases. There should be strong suspicion about the role of infections in any new pelvic symptoms that women develop, especially if they are sexually active. Young, sexually active women sometimes show exposure to several stealth germs such as chlamydia, human papillomavirus, and cytomegalovirus even in the absence of the more commonly known sexually transmitted diseases, such as gonorrhea. Empiric treatment is often a reasonable measure, for low-grade infection within the fallopian tubes is frequently difficult to prove.

Painful Cramping with Menstrual Periods May Indicate Low-grade Pelvic Infection

Symptom: painful periods, persistent pains in the region of the ovaries

Descriptive Diagnosis: menstrual cramping

Actual Diagnosis: pelvic inflammatory disease

Stealth Infection: pelvic infection with chlamydia, anaerobes

Tests to Consider: cultures for chlamydia and other infections

Potential Treatment: various antibiotics; consider empiric treatment

Case in Point: Some women develop nonspecific pelvic discomfort after becoming sexually active. Some of the discomfort may be persistent. Additionally, they may begin to have significantly more cramping with periods than they used to. Sometimes pelvic cultures are done during annual pelvic examinations, and may or may not prove a particular infectious organism. After empiric treatment with antibiotics aimed at pelvic bacteria, the symptoms may improve considerably, or resolve. Often, the resolution of symptoms is the primary clue, and indirect proof, that an infection was present. It is important to protect against reinfection, otherwise the problem will often return.

Persistent Lower Abdominal Pains May Indicate Chronic Pelvic Infection

Symptom: persistent lower abdominal discomfort

Descriptive Diagnosis: nonspecific pelvic pains, irritable bowel syndrome

Actual Diagnosis: pelvic inflammatory disease

Stealth Infection: chlamydia, various organisms

Tests to Consider: cultures at the time of pelvic examination

Potential Treatment: antibacterial antibiotics

Case in Point: A 50-year-old woman had complained of persistent right lower abdominal discomfort for a couple of years; these symptoms were not related to her bowels or her bladder. She had regular Pap smear tests, pelvic exams, and even a colonoscopy and CT scan of the abdomen (all negative). Nor did she have a history of irritable bowel syndrome or other gastrointestinal complaints. Nonetheless, her doctor suspected she had low-grade salpingitis—infection in the tubes leading to the ovaries. She was treated with a brief course of antibiotics, and her symptoms promptly and permanently resolved.

Vaginal Discharge Caused by Pelvic Bacteria Not Responsive to Yeast Creams

Symptom: vaginal discharge, not responsive to creams

Descriptive Diagnosis: vaginitis, yeast infection

Actual Diagnosis: bacterial vaginosis or vaginal trichomoniasis

Stealth Infection: *Gardenella vaginalis*, *Trichomonas vaginalis*, chlamydia

Tests to Consider: cultures at the time of pelvic examination

Potential Treatment: antibiotics, sometimes given empirically

Case in Point: An older patient was told she has atrophic vaginitis due to old age. However, vaginal irritation cleared up with the antibiotic metronidazole. Bacterial vaginosis may complicate pelvic symptoms attributed to menopause or aging processes. Bacterial vaginosis or trichomoniasis may be present in younger women who also have a yeast infection. Treatment of the bacterial infection along with the yeast infection is necessary.

Sores Near Pelvic Opening or Inside Vagina and Sexually Transmitted Diseases

Symptom: recurrent irritation or sores near vaginal opening

Descriptive Diagnosis: yeast infection, bacterial vaginosis

Actual Diagnosis: vaginitis due to sexually transmitted disease

Stealth Infection: herpes simplex, syphilis caused by *Treponema pallidum*, chancroid caused by *Hemophilus ducreyi*.

Tests to Consider: cultures, smears, or blood tests for suspected organisms

Potential Treatment: antibiotics

Case in Point: A young woman sometimes seeks treatment for a "yeast infection" because friends led her to believe that a yeast infection is what her symptoms indicated. Sometimes she will self-treat with a yeast cream, and eventually the sores that bothered her resolve. In such a case it is important to carefully note the history of the symptoms and to consider testing for the above-mentioned sexually transmitted stealth infections, which may require different treatment. It should be noted that the sores of herpes and syphilis will clear up without treatment, but will have significant future consequences unless treated properly.

Head Symptoms

See also section on Brain and Psychiatric Conditions, and Neurological and Nervous Conditions.

The brain is susceptible to several stealth infections, and these are described in the sections noted above. Infections of the ear, nose, throat, and mouth are also discussed in separate sections. Other conditions to consider include the following.

Chronic Sinus Infection Causing Malaise

Symptom: malaise, low-grade headache

Descriptive Diagnosis: chronic fatigue syndrome, sinus congestion

Actual Diagnosis: bacterial sinus infection

Stealth Infection: various bacteria colonizing the sinuses

Tests to Consider: CT scan of sinuses, culture of sinuses or nasal passages

Potential Treatment: various antibiotics

Case in Point: Ten percent or more of the elderly have evidence of sinus infection. The only symptom in some persons is malaise. There may not be a feeling of sinus pain nor nasal stuffiness. When the sinus infection is treated with antibiotics, the generalized feeling of malaise improves.

Shingles of the Head and Face Caused by Herpes zoster

Symptom: sudden-onset pain over part of the face or head

Descriptive Diagnosis: migraine headache, trigeminal neuralgia, temporal arteritis, temporomandibular joint problem

Actual Diagnosis: prodrome to shingles

Stealth Infection: Herpes zoster

Tests to Consider: none necessary, though fluid from the evolving blisters will show the virus

Potential Treatment: antiviral medications against *Varicella-zoster*

Case in Point: *Varicella-zoster*, the chicken pox virus, can linger in the system for decades, then erupt on any surface of the body, including the head, face, or neck, without any warning. The first symptom is usually significant, sometimes severe pain on one side of the head or face. The pain is often attributed to migraine headache, sinus infection, trigeminal neuralgia, temporal arteritis, or other causes. If the skin blisters, which are the main clue to the diagnosis of shingles, erupt in the hair-covered areas, the diagnosis may be missed entirely. Postherpetic neuralgia caused by shingles can be a significant source of persistent head discomfort.

Heart and Cardiovascular Conditions

In recent years inflammation has been found to play a significant role in cardiovascular and circulatory "events," including heart attacks and strokes. Inflammation appears to play a role in destabilizing cholesterol plaques within the arteries. The unstable plaques may cause sudden blockages to occur in coronary arteries or arteries supplying the brain. Inflammatory markers such as C-reactive protein have been found to indicate an increased risk for cardiovascular problems and events.

The possible role of chlamydia, cytomegalovirus, *H. pylori*, and herpes simplex in the development of atherosclerosis is under consideration. Dental disease, particularly gum infection, is being linked to atherosclerosis. Unfortunately, some studies indicate that, despite their role, treatment of these infections may not alter the course of established cardiovascular disease. Further investigations into the role of stealth infections in cardiovascular disease are ongoing.

Chlamydia pneumoniae *Linked to Atherosclerosis and Coronary Disease*

Symptom: findings of coronary or carotid disease, which may or may not have caused a heart attack, angina, or a stroke

Descriptive Diagnosis: atherosclerotic vascular disease

Actual Diagnosis: atherosclerosis compounded by infection

Stealth Infection: *Chlamydia pneumoniae*

Tests to Consider: blood serology tests for chlamydia

Potential Treatment: antibiotics

Case in Point: A 60-year-old school administrator develops angina and undergoes coronary bypass surgery. His recovery is slow. Even several weeks after surgery he has a high sedimentation rate and elevated C-reactive protein, markers of inflammation. Based on serum tests and given evidence that chlamydia might be linked to athero-sclerosis, antibiotics are prescribed. After antibiotics, the patient's sedimentation rate, anemia, and C-reactive proteins gradually normalize.

Severe Sudden Enlargement of the Heart Linked to Virus Infections

Symptom: sudden onset reduced endurance, shortness of breath upon exertion, enlarged heart seen on X-ray with no history of a heart attack or high blood pressure

Descriptive Diagnosis: idiopathic cardiomyopathy

Actual Diagnosis: cardiomyopathy triggered by virus infection

Stealth Infection: parvovirus B19, enterovirus, adenovirus (suspected)

Tests to Consider: blood serology

Potential Treatment: none

Case in Point: On occasion otherwise healthy persons without signs of cardiovascular disease or high cholesterol develop a rapidly progressive enlargement of the heart and congestive heart failure. Parvovirus B19 infection has been reported to be the cause of such idiopathic cardiomyopathy in 51 percent of cases. Enterovirus has been reported to be the cause of idiopathic cardiomyopathy in 9 percent of cases, and adenovirus the cause in 1.6 percent of cases.

Heart Valve Infections Caused by Bacterial Endocarditis

Symptom: shortness of breath, weakness, fatigue

Descriptive Diagnosis: heart valve infections, bacterial endocarditis

Actual Diagnosis: bacterial endocarditis

Stealth Infection: enterococcus, streptococcus, staphylococcus, *Propionibacterium acnes*, periodontal bacteria

Potential Treatment: various antibiotics for extended periods

Case in Point: Enterococcus bacteria can cause bacterial endocarditis. *Propionibacterium acnes* (acne bacteria) has been implicated in heart valve infections. *Staphylococcus aureus*, which normally colonizes the nose, has been linked to subacute bacterial endocarditis. If you have chronic valvular disease you should take antibiotics prior to procedures such as dental work, in order to prevent the circulating periodontal bacteria from gaining a foothold on abnormal valve surfaces of the heart.

Rheumatic Fever and Rheumatic Heart Disease

Symptom: shortness of breath, reduced endurance, fatigue

Descriptive Diagnosis: rheumatic heart disease

Actual Diagnosis: rheumatic heart disease caused by inadequately treated strep infection

Stealth Infection: Group A streptococcus, strep throat

Tests to Consider: throat culture, blood cultures

Potential Treatment: antibiotics against streptococci

Case in Point: Rheumatic fever and rheumatic heart disease are less common in developed countries than a few decades ago, due to prompt antibiotic treatment of throat and other infections caused by streptococci. However, delayed treatment of strep throat or scarlet fever in underdeveloped areas may result in rheumatic heart disease, which damages the valves or the inside lining of the heart. There are still many elderly persons alive today who are receiving treatment for heart damage caused by childhood strep infection. One of the most important reasons for prompt treatment of strep throat with antibiotics is to prevent this potentially severe complication caused by the infection.

Atherosclerosis Linked to Viruses and Other Organisms

Symptom: signs and symptoms of cardiovascular disease

Descriptive Diagnosis: atherosclerosis (hardening of the arteries)

Actual Diagnosis: atherosclerosis compounded by infection

Stealth Infection: cytomegalovirus, herpesviruses, periodontal organisms, *Helicobacter pylori*

Tests to Consider: serum tests for above organisms

Potential Treatment: various antibiotics and antivirals

Case in Point: The above organisms have been suspected to contribute to the development of atherosclerosis, including hardening of the carotid and coronary arteries. However, there is no evidence so far that treatment aimed at these organisms alters the process of atherosclerosis that is linked to their presence.

Inflammatory Abdominal Aortic Aneurysm Linked to Infections

Symptom: none, or some abdominal discomfort

Descriptive Diagnosis: abdominal aortic aneurysm (inflammatory)

Actual Diagnosis: abdominal aortic aneurysm compounded by infection

Stealth Infection: *Chlamydia pneumoniae*, cytomegalovirus

Tests to Consider: abdominal ultrasound, serum tests for the above organisms

Potential Treatment: conventional treatment for abdominal aortic aneurysm

Case in Point: Aneurysms of the aorta are commonly attributed to atherosclerosis or to an inborn weakness of the elastic supports within the aorta. However, recent evidence suggests that inflammation within the wall of the aorta caused by certain infectious organisms may be an equally important cause. There is no evidence yet that treatment of the possible causative organisms alters the progression of the aneurysm.

Kidneys and Stealth Infections

Glomerulonephritis, an inflammatory condition of the kidneys, is caused by one's own immune system, which attacks the kidneys. Infection is not evident, but it is believed that certain infectious organisms, including streptococcus and hepatitis B, may be the hit-and-run triggers of this autoimmune reaction. Rejection of transplanted kidneys may also be triggered by activation of a dormant polyomavirus. Chronic infection of the teeth and gums has recently been correlated with progressive deterioration of kidney function.

Periodontal Disease and Progressive Deterioration of Kidney Function

Symptom: none; laboratory evidence of deteriorating kidney function

Descriptive Diagnosis: progressive renal insufficiency

Actual Diagnosis: progressive renal insufficiency triggered by infection

Stealth Infection: periodontal bacteria

Tests to Consider: dental examination

Potential Treatment: conventional treatment of gum infection

Case in Point: Periodontal disease may accelerate atherosclerosis, which can lead to renal insufficiency. In addition, inflammatory reactions associated with periodontitis may cause direct cellular damage to the microscopic structure of the kidneys and trigger host responses that lead to glomerulonephritis in susceptible persons.

Glomerulonephritis, a Post-infectious Condition Related to Various Organisms

Symptom: progressive renal failure

Descriptive Diagnosis: renal insufficiency due to glomerulonephritis

Actual Diagnosis: glomerulonephritis triggered by infection

Stealth Infection: streptococcus, hepatitis B, various viruses, fungi, and/or rickettsiae

Tests to Consider: serum tests for the above organisms

Potential Treatment: specific anti-infectives against the above organisms

Case in Point: Various infectious agents are known to trigger the autoimmune condition called glomerulonephritis. Once the process has started, treatment of the triggering organism may not be fully effective. However, prompt and early treatment of suspected infections with the above organisms is worthwhile.

Kidney Transplant Rejection

Symptom: none–laboratory evidence of rejection of a recently received transplanted kidney

Descriptive Diagnosis: rejection of kidney transplant

Actual Diagnosis: polyomavirus infection causing rejection of transplanted kidney

Stealth Infection: polyomavirus

Tests to Consider: urine test or blood specimen

Potential Treatment: none for the virus; conventional treatment for transplant rejection

Case in Point: Human polyomavirus has been observed to be associated with rejection of renal transplants. The virus usually becomes activated six to twelve months after transplant. Polyomavirus in the human body is very common; about 90 percent of people are asymptomatic, passive carriers, usually since childhood. When the immune system is suppressed by anti-rejection drugs following kidney transplant, the virus may begin to replicate inside the kidney and may injure the transplanted kidney.

Liver and Hepatitis

The identification of hepatitis C has been a significant event in the understanding of stealth infections. The existence of so-called non-A, non-B hepatitis viruses had been suspected and known for many years. The definite identification of hepatitis C in 1989 led to improved understanding of the many significant health conditions, including liver cancer, caused by this virus.

Infections of the liver by hepatitis viruses are a significant worldwide health problem. More is known about hepatitis A and B than about hepatitis C. Hepatitis B, which is endemic in Southeast Asia, can cause liver cancer. Vaccines against hepatitis A and hepatitis B are available, and have been a major breakthrough in prevention. There is no vaccine for hepatitis C currently. One of the curious properties of the hepatitis C virus is that it can cause a wide range of inflammatory reactions not directly involving the liver, including rheumatological symptoms, kidney problems, and vascular problems.

Low-grade Elevation of Liver Chemistry Tests in Person Who Feels Healthy May Be Due to Hepatitis C

Symptom: none

Descriptive Diagnosis: elevated liver chemistries and enzymes, fatty liver

Actual Diagnosis: hepatitis C infection

Stealth Infection: hepatitis C

Tests to Consider: blood antibody and antigen tests

Potential Treatment: antiviral medication and immunotherapy

Case in Point: For many years, only hepatitis A and B were identified, and hepatitis C was an unknown cause of inflammation of the liver. When present in the liver over time, hepatitis C causes cirrhosis and later even cancer of the liver, often without apparent symptoms other than minor fatigue and malaise. One of the dangers of hepatitis C is dual infection: in patients who also acquire HIV infection, concurrent hepatitis C infection increases the chance of developing hepatocellular cancer five-fold, and multiplies the chance of cirrhosis ten- to twenty-fold. In patients who have schistosomiasis and also hepatitis C, the schistosomiasis will progress more rapidly.

Hepatitis B Causes Cirrhosis of the Liver

Symptom: none, or signs of cirrhosis of the liver

Descriptive Diagnosis: cirrhosis of the liver

Actual Diagnosis: hepatitis B infection

Stealth Infection: hepatitis B

Tests to Consider: blood antigen and antibody tests

Potential Treatment: immunotherapy available

Case in Point: Hepatitis B is a cause of cirrhosis and cancer of the liver. For many years, it may cause only low-grade elevation of liver chemistries. In Southeast Asia, chronic hepatitis B infection is a significant cause of liver problems and liver cancer.

Cancer of the Liver Related to Hepatitis B and C

Symptom: signs and symptoms of liver cancer

Descriptive Diagnosis: cancer of the liver

Actual Diagnosis: cancer of liver due to long-standing hepatitis B or C infection

Stealth Infection: heptatitis B or C

Tests to Consider: serum tests for hepatitis B and C

Potential Treatment: conventional treatment for liver cancer

Case in Point: In persons receiving little regular medical care, cancer of the liver may be the first sign of having carried the hepatitis B or C viruses over many decades.

Spots on the Liver on X-ray Due to Prior Fungal Infection That May Later Reactivate

Symptom: none

Descriptive Diagnosis: granulomatous spots on the liver and spleen

Actual Diagnosis: histoplasmosis or coccidioidomycosis carrier state

Stealth Infection: *Histoplasma capsulatum*, or *Coccidioides immites*

Tests to Consider: skin tests, serum tests

Potential Treatment: antifungal medicines

Case in Point: On occasion, an X-ray or CT scan of the abdomen done for unrelated reasons shows granulomatous spots on the liver. Such spots are indications of prior exposure to the above-noted fungal organisms. If such a person were to undergo chemotherapy or immune-suppressant therapy, the hidden infection may reactivate, causing an infection that arises from within.

Lung and Pulmonary Conditions
See also section on Mouth and Throat.
Stealth infections can enter the body through the lungs. Tuberculosis and infections caused by fungal spores can turn into stealth infections by

going into a dormant state, only to reactivate later when the body's defenses are compromised.

Other organisms that cause chronic infections in the lungs may not be readily identified, because they may not grow readily in the routinely used culture media in the laboratory. Chronic cough attributed to ordinary bronchitis is sometimes caused by *Mycobacterium avium*, a noncurable infection. Other times, persistent bronchitis is caused by psittacosis, transmitted by birds kept in the home as pets.

Chronic Bronchitis Nonresponsive to Ordinary Antibiotics Due to Mycobacterium avium

Symptom: chronic productive cough that does not clear up with regular antibiotics

Descriptive Diagnosis: chronic bronchitis, bronchiectasis

Actual Diagnosis: *Mycobacterium avium-intracellulare* (MAI)

Stealth Infection: *Mycobacterium avium*

Tests to Consider: sputum culture specific for tuberculous organisms

Potential Treatment: clarithromycin, antituberculous antibiotics

Case in Point: This is a condition that may occur in middle-aged persons. Symptoms of bronchitis may be present for months or years before proper diagnosis. Repeated courses of antibiotics may be given, with little benefit. Fortunately MAI is not contagious to others, but it can cause progressive lung injury.

Pulmonary Fibrosis in People Exposed to Birds Caused by Psittacosis

Symptom: cough, shortness of breath

Descriptive Diagnosis: chronic bronchitis, bronchiectasis, asthmatic bronchitis

Actual Diagnosis: psittacosis

Stealth Infection: *Chlamydophila psittaci*

Tests to Consider: blood or sputum tests for psittacosis

Potential Treatment: antibiotics specific for psittacosis

Case in Point: A woman complained to her doctor of pulmonary symptoms, including long-standing shortness of breath. She had a high sedimentation rate, indicative of inflammation, and was diagnosed with pulmonary fibrosis and asthma. In taking her medical history, it was noted that she used to keep parrots as pets, and therefore psittacosis was considered as a possible explanation for her symptoms. Testing confirmed the presence of psittacosis. After taking doxycycline her asthma and pulmonary fibrosis resolved.

Frequently Recurring Lung Infections Related to Poorly Maintained Teeth

Symptom: recurrent bronchitis, persistent cough, gum disease

Descriptive Diagnosis: chronic bronchitis, pneumonia or lung abscess

Actual Diagnosis: pneumonia or lung abscess caused by gum bacteria

Stealth Infection: gum bacteria

Tests to Consider: sputum cultures, dental examination

Potential Treatment: vigorous treatment of gum infection and dental problems

Case in Point: Bacteria harbored in dental plaque can predispose to various lung infections including pneumonia. Poor oral health has been related to the exacerbations of chronic obstructive pulmonary disease (COPD).

Severe Worsening of Asthma Due to Aspergillus Fungus

Symptom: persistent cough, abnormal chest X-ray

Descriptive Diagnosis: chronic asthmatic bronchitis

Actual Diagnosis: pulmonary aspergillosis

Stealth Infection: *Aspergillus fumigatus*

Tests to Consider: sputum culture, biopsy, blood tests

Potential Treatment: antifungals, but only if there is evidence of invasive infection; conventional treatment of asthma.

Case in Point: A patient with chronic asthma and lung infection has a sputum sample tested and cultures are grown. They show evidence of the aspergillus fungus. There is also evidence on blood testing that the body is reacting to the infection. In some cases, the fungus is simply confined to the surface of the lung and windpipe, and no treatment is recommended. In such cases, over time, the fungal colonies often resolve. In this patient's case, the aspergillus fungus actually invaded the lung tissues and required antifungal treatment.

New-onset Asthma, Which Later Becomes Chronic, Triggered by Respiratory Syncytial Virus

Symptom: asthmatic wheezing and cough

Descriptive Diagnosis: asthma

Actual Diagnosis: respiratory syncytial virus infection with bronchospasm

Stealth Infection: respiratory syncytial virus (RSV)

Tests to Consider: test for RSV

Potential Treatment: treatment with anti-RSV neutralizing antibodies available

Case in Point: A 75-year-old typist with a long history of smoking develops a respiratory infection and suffers an acute asthma attack. She is treated for those symptoms. In addition, she is tested for respiratory syncytial virus, which is found to be the cause of her new-onset asthma attack. Viral and possibly mycoplasma infections can trigger acute asthma attacks. There is also evidence that exposure to certain infections during childhood can be a trigger for persistent asthma, though early viral infections may have a protective effect, too. Recent reports suggest that bacterial colonization of the airway in neonates may be one source of persistent asthma in children.

Spots on Chest X-ray Caused by Fungal Stealth Infections That May Reactivate

Symptom: none

Descriptive Diagnosis: granuloma on lung X-ray

Actual Diagnosis: coccidioidomycosis, histoplasmosis, or blastomycosis

Stealth Infection: *Coccidiodes immites, Histoplasma capsulatum, Blastomyces dermatitidis*

Tests to Consider: skin test, serum test

Potential Treatment: antifungal medicines

Case in Point: A 28-year-old woman had a one-month history of swelling of one arm. There were no fever, chills, or signs of infection. X-ray revealed a mediastinal mass, which was proven by biopsy to be caused by histoplasma.

Hidden Tuberculosis Infection That May Reactivate

Symptom: none

Descriptive Diagnosis: granuloma on lung X-ray

Actual Diagnosis: tuberculosis carrier state

Stealth Infection: Mycobacterium tuberculosis

Tests to Consider: skin test

Potential Treatment: antituberculous antibiotics

Case in Point: An elderly patient was treated with prednisone for a rheumatologic problem. He developed swelling of a wrist. The swelling was persistent despite anti-inflammatory medicines. Eventually, fluid from the joint was aspirated and the joint was biopsied. The biopsy revealed tuberculosis, to which he was exposed as a child from a family member who died of the infection. The only other clue over the years to his prior exposure was the long-standing "spot" on his chest x-ray.

Male Genitals and Prostate

See also sections on Urinary Tract and Bladder Conditions and also Gynecologic and Pelvic Conditions.

The male prostate is a spongy structure deep inside the perineum near the bladder outlet and just in front of the rectum. Urinary and sexually transmitted infections can colonize the prostate. From there infection can spread to the nearby spermatic cords, causing epididymitis. Symptoms may or may not be present, but there could be burning on urination or pressure near the rectum. Sometimes the only finding is a few pus cells in the urine and an elevated prostate-specific antigen (PSA) test.

Recent evidence suggests that some cases of cancer of the prostate may be partly related to prior infections, including one particular viral infection and possibly gonorrhea. Venereal warts can infect the penis, and may be transmitted to female sexual partners, in whom they can lead to cancer of the cervix.

Chronic Prostatitis in Men

Symptom: none; occasional rectal discomfort, urinary burning; few pus cells are found on routine urine testing

Descriptive Diagnosis: chronic prostatitis

Actual Diagnosis: bacterial or chlamydia prostatitis

Stealth Infection: chlamydia, various other bacteria

Tests to Consider: urine culture or culture of the urethra, specifically for chlamydia

Potential Treatment: even if cultures are negative, consider empiric treatment with antibiotics; men with Reiter's syndrome may not be cured by antibiotics, but they can still be contagious if they harbor an infectious organism and should be treated

Case in Point: A middle-aged man had frequent, recurrent low-grade prostate infections with some burning and urgency on urination. A short course of antibiotics would usually help. He also had some joint symptoms and eventually a positive HLA-B27 test suggested that he had Reiter's syndrome. After cultures were taken, he was treated with an antibiotic for several months, after which he had no further flare-up of his prostate symptoms over several years of follow-up. Whereas simple bladder infections may be cured with a few-day course of antibiotics, long-standing prostate infections require much longer treatment. Most often the patient's sex partner also needs to be treated at the same time in order to prevent an infection from being passed back and forth.

Prostate Cancer Rarely Due to Gonorrhea

Symptom: symptoms and findings of prostate cancer

Descriptive Diagnosis: prostate cancer

Actual Diagnosis: prostate cancer

Stealth Infection: *Neisseria gonorrhoeae*

Tests to Consider: culture of urine and the urethra

Potential Treatment: usual treatments for the cancer; if there is still active colonization of the prostate with gonorrhea, it should be treated

Case in Point: Although it has not been shown that gonorrhea directly causes prostate cancer, it is suspected that the inflammatory effect of the gonorrhea infection may trigger preexisting cancerous cells to multiply. One survey indicated that the odds of developing prostrate cancer are increased 2.5-fold in men with more than twenty-five lifetime sexual partners, compared with men without such exposure.

Prostate Cancer Linked to Retrovirus

Symptom: those of prostate cancer

Descriptive Diagnosis: prostate cancer

Actual Diagnosis: prostate cancer

Stealth Infection: xenotropic murinelike retrovirus

Tests to Consider: no test currently available

Potential Treatment: none available for the virus; usual treatments for the cancer

Case in Point: This virus is suspected to contribute to the development of prostate cancer in individuals with certain genetic susceptibilities.

Nonspecific Urethritis Caused by Chlamydia

Symptom: burning when urinating, some urethral discharge; urine test and culture are repeatedly negative for bacteria

Descriptive Diagnosis: nosnpecific urethritis

Actual Diagnosis: chlamydia infection

Stealth Infection: *Chlamydia trachomatis*

Tests to Consider: culture specific for chlamydia

Potential Treatment: treatment with antibiotics specific for chlamydia; avoid re-exposure; may need to treat partner

Case in Point: Men who have urinary symptoms may simply ask for a urine test, and when the urine test comes back negative, it is assumed that they don't have an infection that requires treatment. It should be noted that there are many potentially dangerous organisms that do not grow easily on routine cultures, yet are readily treatable with antibiotics (Chlamydia, Lyme disease, Legionnaires' disease are examples). Remember, diagnoses are not based on a single test, but on the combined information gained from a medical history, examination, test results, and other clues. Empiric treatment is sometimes required if direct proof of a highly suspected infection cannot be obtained.

Skin Sores on the Penis Due to Syphilis

Symptom: skin sores on penis that clear up without treatment

Descriptive Diagnosis: chancre, boil, pimple, or minor skin cut

Actual Diagnosis: syphilis

Stealth Infection: *Treponema pallidum*

Tests to Consider: blood test for syphilis, other sexually transmitted diseases

Potential Treatment: antibiotics

Case in Point: Skin sores on the penis of sexually active men need to be considered seriously and with caution. Many conditions can cause such skin sores, including syphilis, herpes, and others. Most often the sores heal despite the continued presence of the stealth germ in the patient's system. Blood tests for infections may not turn positive at the time the sores are present, only at a later time, and cultures of the sore often falsely grow skin organisms and are not fully reliable. Persons with genital sores should have a thorough evaluation.

Penis Sores Due to Herpesvirus and Other Infectious Organisms

Symptom: sores on the penis that clear up without treatment

Descriptive Diagnosis: transient skin sores, boil, chafed skin

Actual Diagnosis: genital herpes infection or chancroid

Stealth Infection: herpes simplex virus type 1 or 2, or *Haemophilus ducreyi*

Tests to Consider: sampling of the skin blister to test for herpesvirus and other microbes

Potential Treatment: antiviral medicines used against herpes and antibiotics against other microbes

Case in Point: Herpes simplex viruses, as well as other infections such as lymphogranuloma venereum, *Haemophilus ducreyi*, syphilis, or human papillomaviruses can infect the skin on the male genitals. Each of these infections can spread from the genitals to other sites such as pelvis, mouth, throat, skin, and anus if those areas are exposed to organisms carried on, or shed from, the infected skin.

Venereal Warts Can Cause Various Cancers

Symptom: warts along the head of the penis

Descriptive Diagnosis: condyloma, venereal warts

Actual Diagnosis: condyloma, veneral warts caused by human papillomavirus

Stealth Infection: human papillomavirus (HPV)

Tests to Consider: cytology test for the virus

Potential Treatment: topical treatments; no antibiotics or antivirals taken internally are effective

Case in Point: Human papillomavirus is of concern not only to women because of potential cancer of the cervix, but equally for men, including gay men. Skin cancer, cancers of the mouth, throat, nose, and possibly of the anus are being associated with human papillomavirus.

Mouth and Throat

Recent studies have reported associations between oral infections and diabetes, heart disease, and stroke, but sufficient evidence does not yet exist to conclusively conclude that one leads to the other. Since dental problems have been traditionally considered to be in the realm of dentistry, the connection between the teeth, gums, and medical diseases was not seriously investigated until recently.

In the mouth there is a fine line between normal flora and what can be considered to be infection. Over five hundred different strains of bacteria may be present in the oral cavity. Gingivitis is diagnosed when the gums around the teeth turn red and inflamed. What causes gingivitis? Is it just due to excessive bacteria, or does it result from infection of the gums when the gums are injured?

When gums are manipulated during dental cleaning and especially if there is some bleeding, bacteria can enter the blood, usually in small numbers. In an otherwise healthy individual, this does not cause a problem; the body's natural immunity is able to take care of it. However, in those with abnormal heart valves, artificial joints or plates in the body, or reduced immune competence, the bacteria that transiently enter the bloodstream can cause endocarditis, osteomyelitis, or infection of the artificial joints. In this way normal gum bacteria can become stealth germs.

Persistent Sore Throat and Mouth Due to Yeast Infection

Symptom: persistent sore throat that does not clear with antibiotics; white patches on tonsils

Descriptive Diagnosis: pharyngitis, strep throat

Actual Diagnosis: yeast infection

Stealth Infection: *Candida albicans*, monilia, yeast

Tests to Consider: swab and culture

Potential Treatment: antifungal medicines

Case in Point: Younger patients sometimes call the doctor's office to ask for a refill of antibiotics for a persistent "strep throat." However, antibiotics, rather than helping, make the sore throat worse. Eventually the inflamed throat with white patches is correctly diagnosed as a yeast infection precipitated by the repeated courses of antibiotics.

Recurrent Sores in the Mouth and Throat Due to Herpes Simplex Virus

Symptom: recurrent mouth sores or throat eruption not responsive to antibiotics

Descriptive Diagnosis: canker sores, stomatitis, mouth sores

Actual Diagnosis: herpes simplex stomatitis

Stealth Infection: herpes simplex

Tests to Consider: test for herpesvirus

Potential Treatment: antiviral against herpesvirus

Case in Point: Patient complained of recurrent mouth sores after "burning her mouth with salsa." A swab of the sores, and blood titers, however, confirmed recent infection with herpes. Her mouth sores cleared when treated with antiviral medication aimed at herpesviruses. Others may conclude that their recurrent mouth sores are harmless canker sores, whereas the sores are due to transmissible herpesvirus.

Recurrent Sore Throat, Mouth and Throat Irritation in Sexually Active Persons Due to Various Infectious Agents

Symptom: recurrent sore throat and mouth sores in person having oral–genital contact

Descriptive Diagnosis: pharyngitis, stomatitis

Actual Diagnosis: herpes simplex stomatitis, or other infectious stomatitis

Stealth Infection: herpes simplex, various organisms

Tests to Consider: culture, swab

Potential Treatment: oral hygiene, antibiotics, antivirals

Case in Point: Oral–genital contact may be a source of the transmission of various organisms, which may cause unexpected sores or eruptions. Head and neck cancers are being attributed to human papillomavirus, formerly confined to the female pelvis and male genitalia. Herpes simplex virus types 1 and 2, formerly confined to their respective regions, can be found interchangeably in either region.

Lichen Planus of the Mouth Caused by Herpesvirus

Symptom: white patches on the inside of the mouth

Descriptive Diagnosis: lichen planus

Actual Diagnosis: lichen planus triggered by virus infection

Stealth Infection: herpesviruses, hepatitis C

Tests to Consider: usual tests for above organisms

Potential Treatment: antivirals specific for herpesviruses, treatment for Hepatitis C.

Case in Point: A middle-aged woman was diagnosed to have lichen planus in her mouth. She also had a history of herpes simplex and was treated with an antiviral for her herpes simplex eruptions. After the treatment began, her lichen planus improved substantially. There is preliminary evidence that lichen planus may be related to Human Herpesvirus 7. There is also a reported association between lichen planus and hepatitis C carrier state.

Muscles

Muscles appear to be resistant to stealth organisms. Inflammatory conditions of the muscles can result from certain infections, such as acute viral influenza, however, influenza does not act as a stealth organism in that case. Invasion of the muscles by the trichinosis organism, usually ingested as part of contaminated pork meat, is a significant issue worldwide in areas where there is poor sanitation.

Trichinosis from Pork in Regions with Poor Sanitation

Symptom: fever, muscle aches, and weakness after eating undercooked meat, especially pork

Descriptive Diagnosis: myositis (muscle inflammation), fibromyalgia

Actual Diagnosis: trichinosis

Stealth Infection: *Trichinella spiralis*

Tests to Consider: serum test

Potential Treatment: none

Case in Point: Trichinosis affects millions of people worldwide, though most cases are asymptomatic. Malaise and muscle aches (in 90 percent) and weakness (in 80 percent) often follow infection, which starts with fever and swelling.

Neurological and Nervous Conditions

See also section on Brain and Psychiatric Conditions.

Stealth infections are rarely the ongoing cause of neurological problems but may be the trigger for many neurodegenerative diseases. As such, treatment of infectious organisms may not be curative after the infection was acquired. On the other hand, prevention of infections that could trigger such neurological conditions may ultimately result in significant public health benefits.

Multiple Sclerosis Linked to Viral Infections

Symptom: symptoms of multiple sclerosis, such as progressive migratory numbness and weakness

Descriptive Diagnosis: multiple sclerosis (MS)

Actual Diagnosis: multiple sclerosis possibly triggered by infection

Stealth Infection: various infectious organisms suspected as triggers

Tests to Consider: blood tests for exposure to the organisms listed below

Potential Treatment: antivirals or antibiotics if coexisting or underlying infection found

Case in Point: A number of viruses and infectious agents have been implicated in causing multiple sclerosis: *Chlamydia pneumoniae*, herpesvirus 6, Epstein–Barr virus, and endogenous retroviruses. Some of these infections have incubation periods of years and may cause remitting and relapsing disease, causing myelin destruction mediated by a variety of mechanisms. Cause and effect is not yet conclusively proven.

Infections Predisposing to Stroke

Symptom: usual symptoms of stroke

Descriptive Diagnosis: stroke

Actual Diagnosis: stroke

Stealth Infection: periodontal infection

Tests to Consider: dental examination

Potential Treatment: thorough treatment of gum and dental infections

Case in Point: *Aggregatibacter actinomycetemcomitans* are periodontal organisms whose presence may increase the likelihood of stroke. Patients with an antibody to this organism were 1.6 times more likely to have a first stroke and 2.6 times more likely to have a secondary stroke.

Sudden Drooping of the Face Due to Bell's Palsy Linked to Viral Trigger

Symptom: sudden-onset drooping of the muscles of one side of the face

Descriptive Diagnosis: Bell's palsy

Actual Diagnosis: Bell's palsy triggered by infection

Stealth Infection: herpesvirus type 1, possibly cytomegalovirus, Epstein-Barr virus

Tests to Consider: blood test for herpesvirus exposure

Potential Treatment: antiviral for herpes

Case in Point: Even though for many years Bell's palsy was thought to be idiopathic, meaning of unknown cause, there is evidence that it may be triggered by underlying infection with one of the herpesviruses, most likely herpes simplex and possibly other infectious organisms. As such, antiviral medicine aimed at herpesviruses has been tried in persons who develop new-onset Bell's palsy. Recent reports indicate little benefit from one particular medicine, acyclovir. Further studies are ongoing.

Rapidly Progressive Paralysis Caused by Guillain-Barré Syndrome Triggered by Infection

Symptom: rapidly progressive paralysis

Descriptive Diagnosis: Guillain-Barré syndrome

Actual Diagnosis: Guillain-Barré syndrome triggered by infection

Stealth Infection: *Campylobacter jejuni*, possibly mycoplasma

Tests to Consider: serum tests for the above organisms

Potential Treatment: conventional treatment for Guillain-Barré syndrome

Case in Point: Guillain-Barré syndrome has been long suspected to have an infectious trigger, but treatment with anti-infectives has not been found to be of benefit. However, signs of infection with the above organisms should be sought, and treatment aimed at eradicating these pathogenic organisms may be useful even if doing so does not directly benefit the neurological problem. Another condition called transverse myelitis may also have an infectious trigger.

Various Infections Causing Loss of Balance, Numbness, and Other Neurological Problems

Symptom: gradual numbness, loss of balance, skin rashes, dementia

Descriptive Diagnosis: tabes dorsalis, neurosyphilis

Actual Diagnosis: neurosyphilis, Lyme disease, Whipple's disease

Stealth Infection: *Treponema pallidum*, *Borrelia burgdorferi*, *Tropheryma whippellii*

Tests to Consider: usual tests for syphilis, Lyme disease, Whipple's disease

Potential Treatment: antibiotics

Case in Point: Various neurological problems may arise from several treatable bacterial organisms, which may give various symptoms, without the presence of fever or other obvious signs of infection. Each of these organisms is a true stealth germ. Long-term infection with any of these can produce the well-described progressive neurodegenerative conditions attributed to each one.

Nose and Sinuses

"Keep your nose clean" is an old adage that is usually interpreted as advice to stay out of trouble. What kind of trouble can your nose get you into? Interestingly, the nose is the location or source of some important stealth infections.

Chronic Irritation Inside the Lining of the Nostrils Caused by Staph, Which Can Lead to Osteomyelitis

Symptom: chronic irritation of the nasal lining and recurrent crusty spots inside the nostrils

Descriptive Diagnosis: allergy, hay fever, vasomotor rhinitis, sinus infection

Actual Diagnosis: staph infection of the nasal passage

Stealth Infection: *Staphylococcus aureus, including MRSA*

Tests to Consider: bacterial culture of the nasal passage

Potential Treatment: mupirocin ointment; combination of strong antibiotics may be needed to fully eradicate the colonies of bacteria

Case in Point: A patient with poor hygiene developed osteomyelitis of the bone in his spine. After successful treatment, he had another similar infection a year later. No outside source of the infection was found, but he had crusty deposits in his nasal passages. These deposits were cultured and grew the same staph organism that was found in his bone. Many patients who are being treated for nasal allergies are found to have colonization of the nasal passages with staph. When the staph is treated with topical ointments or other measures, their nasal sensitivity improves substantially. Methicillin-restistant *Staphylococcus aureus* (MRSA) can be carried and harbored in the nasal passages, and can be the source of MRSA infection which is spread to others, which is especially dangerous to those with compromised immunity.

Recurring Crusty Cold Sore Inside the Nostril Due to Herpesvirus

Symptom: sore spot that periodically returns in a certain location inside the nostrils, then goes away by itself for extended periods of time

Descriptive Diagnosis: pimple or boil inside the nose

Actual Diagnosis: recurrent cold sore due to herpesvirus

Stealth Infection: herpes simplex virus

Tests to Consider: sampling of the blister or boil to test for herpes (or staph)

Potential Treatment: antiviral medicine for herpes

Case in Point: Many persons experience a small sore which is rather tender inside their nostril that flares up on occasion, then goes away. They attribute this to having nicked the spot in their nose while picking it, though they don't remember doing so. Testing may confirm that the spot is a recurrent cold sore due to herpes simplex virus. It is important to know the accurate diagnosis, because the person with the sore in their nose may be contagious to others, especially young children or those with immune problems.

Chronic Sinusitis Causing Headaches

Symptom: persistent sinus pressure and headache despite treatment of sinus infection with antibiotics

Descriptive Diagnosis: sinus headaches

Actual Diagnosis: chronic sinusitis

Stealth Infection: various

Tests to Consider: CT scan of the sinuses; consider nasal culture; ear, nose, and throat (ENT) evaluation

Potential Treatment: extended treatment with antibiotics

Case in Point: Ten percent of the elderly have evidence of sinusitis on CT scans done for other reasons. Many younger persons are also treated for sinus infection and improve transiently, but then their symptoms return. Often the reason is that they were not treated for a long enough period to ensure eradication of the infection. Whereas a simple bladder infection can be cured in three to five days, the necessary length of treatment with antibiotics for a significant sinus infection may be several weeks.

Progressive Bumpy Deformity of the Outside of the Nose Due to Rosacea

Symptom: red bumps on the skin of the nose that are deep enough to begin to distort the form and shape of the nose

Descriptive Diagnosis: boils, pimples, acne

Actual Diagnosis: rhinophyma due to rosacea

Stealth Infection: bacterial or other organism causing the problem has not been proven, but rosacea responds to antibiotics in pill or topical form

Tests to Consider: none

Potential Treatment: metronidazole, doxycycline

Case in Point: Symptoms and findings include bumpy, enlarging nose with prominent pores, some redness, sometimes accompanied by ruddy cheeks or irritation of the eyelids. Early recognition and treatment may prevent a progressive deformity of the shape of the nose. (See also the sections on Stealth Infections and the Skin, and on Eye for other problems caused by rosacea.)

Obesity and Stealth Germs

When thinking about excessive weight gain, most of us attribute it to overeating or family predisposition. In fact, when we are seriously ill with an infection, we often tend to lose weight. A few years ago, it was reported that chickens infected with a particular virus called adenovirus developed excessive intra-abdominal fat but maintained low cholesterol and triglyceride levels. Tests for the same virus in overweight persons confirmed a link described below. There is also some evidence that an imbalance of certain bacteria in the gut may be associated with weight gain.

Obesity Linked to Adenovirus Exposure

Symptom: obesity

Descriptive Diagnosis: obesity

Actual Diagnosis: obesity in part triggered by infection

Stealth Infection: human adenoviruses 36 and 37

Tests to Consider: none, though serum antibody test for the virus is available

Potential Treatment: none; avoid exposure

Case in Point: Evidence of exposure to adenovirus 36 is found in a higher proportion of obese persons than in the general population.

In fact, 15 percent of the obese carry antibodies to adenovirus 36. This virus, along with another strain, adenovirus 37, has been implicated in the obesity of animals including chickens, mice, and primates. Adenoviruses 36 and 37 are transmitted through the air and can cause respiratory infection, cold symptoms, gastrointestinal problems, and conjunctivitis (pinkeye).

Obese patients with exposure have unusually low cholesterol and triglyceride levels despite their obesity. Inoculation into animals of serum from patients who have evidence of active carrier state of the virus (indicated by persons with antibodies developing antibodies against each other's serum) produce predictable fat deposition and lowering of cholesterol and triglycerides. At this time there is no treatment for the virus, nor evidence that treating it would reverse the tendency to become obese. However, avoiding exposure may be one way to reduce the tendency to excessive weight gain.

Obesity Linked to Disproportionate Balance of Bacteria in the Gut

Symptom: obesity

Descriptive Diagnosis: obesity

Actual Diagnosis: obesity in part triggered by infection

Stealth Infection: Firmicutes and Bacteroidetes

Tests to Consider: none

Potential Treatment: none, other than losing weight to restore balance

Case in Point: Numerous groups of beneficial bacteria inhabit the colon. Following observations and studies of obese mice, studies in human beings found that overabundance of the bacteria Firmicutes in relation to Bacteroidetes was present in obese individuals, and the opposite was true in normal-weight persons. Additionally, as the obese individuals lost weight, an increase of the relative abundance of

Bacteriodetes occurred, and significantly correlated to weight loss, despite high calorie intake.

In the laboratory, when the guts of germ-free mice were populated with microbes from the guts of obese mice, they had a significantly greater increase in total body fat (without increase in food consumption) than those receiving microbes from the guts of lean mice. These results suggest that the microbes in the gut may have something to do with the pathophysiology of obesity. No practical treatment or management is available at this time.

Stealth Infections and the Skin

Numerous conditions which are not proven to be due to infection may affect the skin, including eczema, psoriasis, and allergies. Often an infectious component is missed when a new organism invades the same area as another, previously diagnosed condition. Empiric treatment is sometimes useful if an infection is believed to complicate a noninfectious chronic skin condition. Exhaustive lists of infectious skin conditions, too numerous to list here, can be found in textbooks of dermatology.

Erythema Nodosum Linked to Various Infections

Symptom: red bumps under the skin along the shins

Descriptive Diagnosis: erythema nodosum

Actual Diagnosis: erythema nodosum due to underlying infection

Stealth Infection: in children, streptococcus; in adults, strep; bowel infections with tuberculosis, *Yersinia enterocolitica*, salmonella, campylobacter; lung infection with *Mycoplasma pneumoniae*, tuberculosis, sexually transmitted infection with Lymphogranuloma venereum

Tests to Consider: culture stools or sputum, blood test for mycoplasma

Potential Treatment: specific antibiotic depending on the organism

Case in Point: This is a common condition, usually affecting younger adults, more often women than men. It shows up a few weeks after an infection or other event, and may cause fever and achiness along with the tender nodules under the skin. Diagnosis is sometimes not correctly made.

Seborrheic Dermatitis Due to Malassezia ovale

Symptom: dandrufflike eruption on the scalp, face, or chest

Descriptive Diagnosis: seborrheic dermatitis, dandruff

Actual Diagnosis: seborrheic dermatitis caused in part by fungal infection

Stealth Infection: Malassezia ovale

Tests to Consider: none necessary

Potential Treatment: antifungal medicines

Case in Point: A 78-year-old man had a long history of eczema over much of his body diagnosed by dermatologists. This was treated with regular application of cortisone-containing creams. He has also had some dandruff on his scalp and eyebrows. Over the past few years, his skin condition has worsened and he has had uncomfortable itching and flaking of the skin on his chest, face, and head. His internist diagnosis, seborrheic dermatitis on his scalp and his chest. The doctor was aware that this condition is caused by a skin fungus and can respond to a particular antifungal medicine. After several weeks on the prescribed medicine, the patient's overall skin condition, including the previously widespread eczema, improved more than 90 percent.

Acne Bacteria Implicated in Various Conditions

Symptom: various problems, see below

Descriptive Diagnosis: acne

Actual Diagnosis: acne due to infection with propinobacterium

Stealth Infection: *Propionibacterium acnes*

Tests to Consider: none

Potential Treatment: antibiotics specific for the organism

Case in Point: *Propionibacterium acnes* causes acne but has recently been implicated in certain chronic diseases. It is being linked to heart valve infection, postoperative infection or failure of implanted orthopedic prostheses, and possibly to inflammatory sciatica.

Lyme Disease with Skin Eruption

Symptom: skin rash following tick bite, followed by arthritic symptoms

Descriptive Diagnosis: erythema chronicum migrans

Actual Diagnosis: Lyme disease, borreliosis

Stealth Infection: *Borrelia burgdorferi*

Tests to Consider: usual test for Lyme disease

Potential Treatment: antibiotics

Case in Point: Erythema chronicum migrans is a rash characteristic of evolving Lyme disease transmitted by tick bites. For more extended discussion see Lyme disease under section on Arthritis and Joints.

Rosy Cheeks Due to Rosacea Respond to Antibiotics

Symptom: rosy cheeks and adult acne

Descriptive Diagnosis: rosacea

Actual Diagnosis: rosacea

Stealth Infection: bacteria or other organisms have not been conclusively identified as the cause of rosacea, but the condition responds to antibiotics both in pill and topical form

Tests to Consider: none

Potential Treatment: antibiotics

Case in Point: Infectious organisms that may cause, trigger, or perpetuate rosacea have not been definitively identified. The skin condition does, however, respond well to certain antibiotics. More important, rosacea can spread onto the eyelids and into the tear ducts, causing dry eye syndrome or plugging of the tear ducts. Extended treatment with antibiotics can alleviate this complication of rosacea.

Viruses and Skin Cancer

Symptom: various skin cancers in persons who have previously been exposed to condyloma warts

Descriptive Diagnosis: skin cancer, nonmelanoma

Actual Diagnosis: skin cancer triggered by papillomavirus

Stealth Infection: human papillomavirus

Tests to Consider: biopsy

Potential Treatment: usual treatment for skin cancer and measures aimed at eradicating the virus from the skin

Case in Point: Human papillomavirus, which has been familiar for many years as the cause of condyloma (venereal warts) is being increasingly found to contribute to cancers on various surfaces of the body. It is linked to skin cancers as well as cancers of the throat and nasal passages, along with its well-known association with cancer of the cervix. This virus is of great interest in investigating the role of viruses in cancer causation, and the prevention of such cancers through vaccination.

Hives Occasionally Associated with Underlying Sinus and Other Infections

Symptom: hives

Descriptive Diagnosis: urticaria (hives)

Actual Diagnosis: hives due to underlying infection

Stealth Infection: sinus infection and other infections

Tests to Consider: X-rays or scans of the sinuses, cultures

Potential Treatment: antibiotics

Case in Point: Hives have been associated with underlying sinus infections. If you have hives, and sinus infection is suspected or proven, taking appropriate antibiotics for the sinus infection may be useful in eradicating one possible underlying factor that perpetuates the hives. Hives have also been associated with other underlying infections, such as staph colonization of the nose, *Helicobacter pylori*, and even *Blastocystis hominis*.

Relapsing and Spreading Sores or Blisters Due to Herpesvirus

Symptom: spreading skin rash in person who may have had cold sores and fever blisters

Descriptive Diagnosis: eczema herpeticum (disseminated herpes)

Actual Diagnosis: disseminated herpes virus infection of skin

Stealth Infection: herpes simplex virus

Tests to Consider: sampling of the skin blister to test for herpesvirus

Potential Treatment: antiviral medicines specific for herpesviruses

Case in Point: After cutting down a large cactus plant, a male patient developed an itchy and burning skin condition ultimately diagnosed as eczema. This was treated for an extended period of time with medicines usually given for eczema. However, the condition was worsening, and the skin was biopsied. The biopsy indicated that the abnormal skin was overrun with the herpes simplex virus. His long-standing "eczema" improved more than 75 percent after treatment with antiviral medication.

Shingles Eruption Due to Chicken Pox Virus

Symptom: sudden-onset pain and sensitivity of a patch of skin over some part of the body, followed a week or so later by clusters of blistering skin eruption

Descriptive Diagnosis: shingles

Actual Diagnosis: *Herpes zoster* virus causing shingles

Stealth Infection: *Varicella zoster / Herpes zoster* virus

Tests to Consider: sampling of the skin blisters to test for the virus

Potential Treatment: antiviral medication

Case in Point: The *Varicella zoster* virus is a classic and prime example of a stealth infection. After getting over a bout with chicken pox during childhood, almost everyone continues to harbor a few leftover organisms of this virus of the herpesvirus family in their body. There is no sign whatsoever in one's system of carrying this virus. However, many decades later, it may re-emerge in virtually any part of the body from the head to the limbs, and cause the classic painful, blistery shingles eruption, then go back into hiding once again, with only a rare second appearance. The currently available shingles vaccine greatly reduces the likelihood of suffering from an eruption of shingles.

Hot Tub Dermatitis Due to Pseudomonas aeruginosa

Symptom: skin bumps thought to be impetigo or insect bites after using a hot tub

Descriptive Diagnosis: insect bites, folliculitis, impetigo

Actual Diagnosis: pseudomonas infection acquired from contaminated water

Stealth Infection: *Pseudomonas aeruginosa*

Tests to Consider: culture abnormal skin spot

Potential Treatment: antibiotic against pseudomonas and decontaminate the hot tub

Case in Point: A woman developed itchy bumps on her skin, which were attributed to insect bites. These "insect bites" were recurring over much of her body, below the neck. Interestingly, this started happening about the same time she began using a hot tub one of her friends recently installed. She was seen at an urgent care clinic, and she was thought to have either insect bites or impetigo, but her skin problem did not improve with treatment given for these conditions. Culture of the skin spots proved the pseudomonas infection.

Stasis Dermatitis and Stasis Ulcerations Complicated by Tinea

Symptom: dry, leathery, rust-colored skin around the ankles, with poorly healing sores.

Descriptive Diagnosis: stasis dermatitis

Actual Diagnosis: tinea colonization of the abnormal skin in addition to stasis dermatitis

Stealth Infection: *Tinea corporis*

Tests to Consider: fungal culture of skin

Potential Treatment: antifungal creams or pills

Case in Point: Also described in the section under feet, this condition usually happens in older persons or in those with chronically swollen ankles. The skin around the ankles becomes dry and develops a rust-colored appearance, and may become hardened and leathery. The skin in the area may also show signs of athlete's foot fungus, and the toenails may show signs of onychomycosis (nail fungus). The skin affected by the athlete's foot fungus often extends into the area of stasis dermatitis. Yet most of the attention is focused on the dermatitis, or on bacteria, and treatment of the fungus infection is often neglected. Treatment of both conditions has to be undertaken at the same time, along with meticulous skin and wound care, in order for the skin to heal.

Urinary Tract and Bladder Conditions

See also sections on and Male Genitals and Prostate and Gynecologic and Pelvic Conditions. Many persons experience urinary symptoms during their lifetime. Burning on urination is common. A pus (white blood cells) or blood in the urine may be noted in otherwise asymptomatic individuals. An unexpected complication of urinary infections in a few susceptible individuals is an arthritic condition called Reiter's syndrome. Some chronic urinary conditions are due to low-grade infections, while other problems such as interstitial cystitis are inflammatory conditions possibly triggered by a hit-and-run infection that is no longer present.

Reactive Arthritis Triggered by Urinary Infection

Symptom: episodic but persistent burning on urination along with arthritic symptoms and sometimes uveitis, an inflammatory condition of the eye

Descriptive Diagnosis: chronic urethritis

Actual Diagnosis: Reiter's syndrome

Stealth Infection: *Chlamydia trachomatis* and others

Tests to Consider: culture of urethra for chlamydia

Potential Treatment: antibiotics

Case in Point: Soon after sexual relations with a new partner, a man develops some burning on urination, but bladder infection is not confirmed. His symptoms continue, along with certain joint pains, and even a flare-up of inflammation in the eye. He may be told that he has recurrent prostate infections. A chromosomal predisposition to the condition is the presence of the HLA-B27 chromosomal marker. Aside from chlamydia, gonorrhea, certain bowel infections with salmonella, shigella, and campylobacter may also trigger the syndrome in susceptible individuals. Prompt treatment with an antibiotic specific for chlamydia or the other triggering germs is warranted, but may not be helpful if started too late.

Tropical Bladder Flukes Later Cause Bladder Cancer

Symptom: recurrent blood in the urine of persons living in or having traveled to tropical countries

Descriptive Diagnosis: hematuria, urinary infection

Actual Diagnosis: schistosomiasis

Stealth Infection: *Schistosoma haematobium*

Tests to Consider: urine or stool tests for the schistosome eggs

Potential Treatment: antihelminthic antimicrobial medicines are available and effective

Case in Point: There may be upward of 200 million persons in the tropics who carry these parasitic worms/flukes, which are common in agricultural areas of Africa, South America, and Asia. Symptoms of schistosomiasis include blood in the urine and burning on urination, with later difficulty in urination. Often there are few symptoms of illness until progressive urinary obstruction occurs. Other flukes related to *Schistosoma haematobium* include *S. japonicum*, *S. mansoni* and *S. mekongi* all of which produce more noticeable illness, including diarrhea.

Interstitial Cystitis Could Be Caused by an Unknown Infectious Organism Not Yet Identified

Symptom: chronic urinary urgency, frequently not responsive to commonly used antibiotics

Descriptive Diagnosis: interstitial cystitis

Actual Diagnosis: bladder infection mimicking interstitial cystitis

Stealth Infection: currently not known, but some researches suspect that interstitial cystitis could be caused by an infectious organism that has not yet been identified

Tests to Consider: cystoscopy and biopsy, bacterial, viral cultures

Potential Treatment: conventional treatment for interstitial cystitis; brief empiric trial treatment with antivirals or antibiotics could be considered with careful attention to any improvement of symptoms

Case in Point: Although no commonly known bacteria, fungi, or viruses are ordinarily found in the urine of patients diagnosed with interstitial cystitis, many researchers believe that it's possible that the condition is caused by an infectious organism that has not yet been identified. Another factor may be an autoimmune reaction of the body against its own bladder tissue, possibly triggered by a hit-and-run infection. Occasionally extended treatment of patients diagnosed with interstitial cystitis with antibiotics aimed at difficult-to-culture organisms such as Chlamydia, results in improvement.

5. Special Conditions

Pregnancy

The topic of infection during pregnancy is a lengthy and complex medical subject. Detailed discussions are best left to the experts, and to textbooks of perinatology, obstetrics, and infectious diseases. I will touch on the subject briefly, because some infections of pregnant women directly involve stealth germs or act similarly to stealth infections.

Worldwide, the unwanted consequences of infections during pregnancy continue to be a serious issue. Such infections still continue to cause problems despite the pioneering work by Ignác Semmelweis. As a result of his efforts promoting hand washing and hygienic medical practices on maternity wards, childbed fever is gone, for the most part. However, pregnant women need to be protected from infections during pregnancy, not just at the time of delivery. The developing fetus is at risk when the mother is exposed to infection and needs similar protection. Perinatology is the field of medicine that deals with such perinatal care and issues.

Women may carry stealth germs prior to becoming pregnant and then continue to harbor these germs throughout their pregnancy. Equally likely, they can be exposed to and acquire new infections during the pregnancy. Pregnancy itself alters the immune system to a degree though, contrary to conventional wisdom, it does not weaken it. Nevertheless, on rare occasion quietly harbored germs reactivate during pregnancy.

Fortunately, many stealth infections carried by women are not directly transmitted to the fetus. For example, there is no proven evidence that the ulcer bacteria, *H. pylori*, or the chicken pox virus, *Varicella zoster*, are transmitted to the fetus during pregnancy. However, there is a very significant likelihood of transmitting other infectious germs. Transmission of the

HIV virus from mother to fetus is a significant problem in areas of the world where this infection is widespread. Mothers carrying syphilis will transmit the treponema organism to the baby. A lesser-known infection called toxoplasmosis is also transmissible in the womb.

The newborn is also vulnerable to infection during birth, resulting from direct contact with germs as he or she exits through the birth canal. As we have already discussed, chlamydia present in the birth canal can enter the eye of the newborn and cause serious eye infections, which can lead to blindness if not treated. Herpesvirus in the birth canal can also infect the new baby. Vaginal and rectal colonization of pregnant women with the staph organism (*Staphylococcus aureus*) is increasingly documented. Some of these organisms are becoming resistant to conventional antibiotics and may be a source of significant problems.

One of the lesser-known germs that can cause an undiagnosed infection during pregnancy is *Listeria monocytogenes*. A pregnant mother may develop a brief spell with chills, fever, and back pain. A urine test done to look for bacterial infection is negative, and the fever and chills subside without specific treatment. Since basic tests are not diagnostic, the infection is usually attributed to an unknown virus. Yet the true cause of the infection is a treatable bacterium that in some cases can have serious adverse effects on the pregnancy.

A virus that can affect pregnant women is parvovirus B19. It can be transmitted from mother to fetus, though fortunately this happens only in a minority of cases. In children, the virus causes so-called "fifth disease," with coldlike symptoms and "slapped cheek" redness of the face. Pregnant women who catch this infection have a 2 to 6 percent risk of losing the pregnancy. The fetus can develop severe anemia, myocarditis (inflammation of the heart muscle), and other complications.

Is there evidence of harm to the fetus from ordinary infections such as colds or bladder infections? Cause and effect is once again very difficult to establish. However, there are certain clues. Mothers of babies born with cerebral palsy frequently report infection during pregnancy. In one survey approximately one-third of such mothers had a significant infection, excluding minor colds, most often infection of the urinary tract. A definite cause-and-effect relationship should not be drawn from this observation, however. Perhaps these mothers have a weaker-than-average immune system or some other minor aberrancy that leads to both problems. Nevertheless, once again we are reminded of the precepts of the ancients, who observed that those who live a life of "purity" (germ-free-ness?) are the most likely to be blessed with good health and healthy children.

Of course, infections are only one of the many health issues that require attention during pregnancy. There is clear evidence that poisonous chemicals, or deliberately taken substances that circulate in the blood of drug-using mothers, can harm the fetus. Making motherhood safe in developing countries is a significant worldwide social problem. If you are pregnant or plan to become pregnant, seek the advice of a professional with expertise in the field of obstetrics. (Please also read the disclaimer at the beginning of this book.)

Fortunately the human species is durable and built for survival. Most pregnancies proceed without complications, and the vast majority of children are born healthy, to the joy of their parents and family. Let us now look briefly at newborn children and certain infections that may affect their development.

Childhood Development

Persons living in the so-called developed countries, especially those with average or better economic means, are fortunate. Their children are likely to remain protected from many infections due to the availability of clean water, uncontaminated food, and access to health care.

In less-developed parts of the world, however, numerous infections are still rampant. They are among the leading causes of developmental disabilities in children who live in these regions. I refer you to sections of the report *The Infectious Etiology of Chronic Diseases* quoted earlier, and to other references on the subject.

Children in many ways are remarkably resilient and durable. They are also vulnerable and largely dependent on their parents. Congenitally acquired infections passed on from the mother to child are a significant problem in the developing world. There is further jeopardy to the newborn from infections lurking in their environment, including contaminated water and food. Many of these infections may affect their developing organ systems, including the senses such as vision and hearing, as well as the nervous system. In the nervous system, chronic low-grade infections can lead to movement/motor problems, seizures, and intellectual, learning, and behavioral disabilities. It is inestimable to what degree such problems are harmful not only to individuals, but to entire societies.

The list of infections and their consequences is virtually endless. The table highlights just some infectious conditions affecting childhood development. Some of these conditions can be devastating, and many result in permanent problems. However, if identified, some of these diseases—syphilis, worm infestation, herpes, and malaria—are treatable. Additionally, recent reports have linked crib death, or SIDS, to hidden infections.

Infectious conditions affecting children are well known to concerned parents, but even more so to public health officials, pediatricians, and other specialists. Agencies such as the United Nations Children's Fund (UNICEF), the World Health Organization (WHO), as well as other organizations and numerous individuals continue to make strident efforts on behalf of the health of the children of the world. These worthwhile causes should be supported. Moreover, each one of us also needs to take direct personal responsibility for our own health and the health of our children.

Animal-borne Infections

In considering exposures from our environment, we also need to think about infections that may come from animals in our midst. Dating back to the earliest days of the human race, human beings have had close association with animals, which were kept as pets or domesticated farm animals. Human-animal associations were in many ways helpful or even essential to our own survival over the millennia.

Many persons continue to take advantage of the benefits of animal companionship. There is evidence that pets provide measurable benefit to

Table 5.
Infections That Affect Childhood Development

Stealth Germ	Observed Result
Treponema pallidum	causes congenital syphilis syndrome
Toxoplasma gondii	causes congenital toxoplasmosis syndrome
rubella virus	causes congenital rubella syndrome
cryptosporidiosis	causes developmental disabilities
helminthic (worm) infestations	cause developmental growth retardation
HIV	leads to various developmental disabilities
herpesvirus	leads to neurodevelopmental disabilities and possibly to schizophrenia
Plasmodium falciparum	organism which causes malaria; causes delayed cognitive development in children and childhood anemia
measles virus	causes developmental disabilities
Borna disease virus	contributes to neurodevelopmental disorders

the well-being of seniors, children, or those who are lonely. Even so, are animals uniformly beneficial to our physical health, or can they also be the source of potentially hazardous infections? One historic example of the potential benefit of the association with animals is the protection of farm children against the serious and deadly human smallpox as a result of their natural exposure to cowpox. However, not all animal-carried infections are similarly beneficial or harmless.

Many animal diseases do not infect humans. However, human beings can become ill from some germs that animals carry without the animal showing signs of illness. To heighten awareness, let us highlight some infections that may spread to human beings through contact with apparently healthy animals who appear to be asymptomatic carriers. Some of these infections are carried by domestic animals in areas of the world where sanitation is poor and water and food supplies are of questionable purity. An unexpected source of germs harmful to humans is antibiotic-treated livestock, which develop and carry antibiotic-resistant bacteria, which may be transmitted to those working with the animals. Other infections can come from household pets such as cats, birds, reptiles, or other exotic pets. Yet others come indirectly from wild animals by ingestion of contaminated meat by hunters, or in the form of deer ticks from wild deer.

In the case of domesticated animals, herd animals such as cattle, goats, and sheep may carry brucella, which causes undulant fever. The organism is transmitted by drinking contaminated milk or eating contaminated meat. Pigs may carry trichinosis, which humans can acquire by eating contaminated pork. Sheep can carry liver flukes. Chickens are one of the sources of the deadly avian influenza (bird flu) and salmonella. Mad cow disease, or bovine spongiform encephalopathy, may be potentially harmful to humans.

Cats may carry campylobacter, *Cryptosporidium*, and *Giardia*, all of which can cause diarrheal illnesses. They can also harbor salmonella, yersinia, and toxoplasmosis. Cat scratch disease is caused by *Bartonella henselae*. Cat bites transmit pasteurella. Pet birds can be the source of psittacosis lung infection, which may cause a persistent asthmalike condition in humans, and also may harbor cryptococcosis. Pet reptiles may carry salmonella.

Deer ticks are the source of Lyme disease and Rocky Mountain spotted fever. Hunters eating the meat of animals carrying the prion-caused chronic wasting disease in deer or elk have been reported to develop spongiform encephalopathy, a rapidly progressive brain disease.

Exotic pets are also potential sources of infection. Hedgehogs and chinchillas can be the source of a skin condition caused by the fungus *Trichophyton mentagrophytes*. This fungus causes an inflammatory skin condition in human beings similar to athlete's foot. Flying squirrels carry *Rickettsia prowazekii*, which causes typhus fever. Gerbils can carry *Giardia lamblia*, which can cause the predictable intestinal condition in humans. Prairie dogs may carry plague, tularemia, and monkeypox. Cockatoos and macaws are hosts for *Cryptococcus neoformans*, a bacteria that may cause significant illness in immunosuppressed patients.

Once again, the list of germs is endless, and details of these conditions are beyond the scope of this book. For more information about such conditions, consult infectious disease textbooks and other references.

As described earlier, throughout our lives we live in a sea of germs, and are covered with layers of germs, but usually we get along with them very well. Practicing basic principles of hygiene generally protects us quite well. There is no question, however, that there are certain infectious germs that can cause greater or lesser amounts of harm. Instead of fear and worry about infections, we should become well informed about our infectious enemies so we can take prudent action against them by protecting ourselves and those around us.

Discovering hidden infections within our systems and protecting ourselves from potential consequences should now be our focus.

6. What Else Could It Be?

What If Your Evaluation Finds "Nothing"?

After reading about the various conditions caused by stealth germs you might be somewhat concerned that you, too, have one hiding in your system. Maybe you've visited your doctor to have your symptoms and concerns evaluated. If a treatable infection was found as a result of the consultation, you likely received appropriate information and treatment.

Suppose you returned for the follow-up visit with your doctor, and you were told that "we found nothing." What does that really mean?

"We Found Nothing" Versus "There Is Nothing"

Clearly there is a difference between "we found nothing (abnormal)" and "there is nothing (abnormal)." In general "we found nothing, so far" means that the screening examinations and tests that were ordered to look for particular conditions yielded negative results at the time they were done. In other words, nothing truly abnormal was found on the examination or on the tests that were chosen to be performed thus far. Clearly, that doesn't prove conclusively that you are not harboring stealth germs in your body, as there is no foolproof test that can find everything. The absence of a large number of possible conditions does not exclude the presence of some other previously undetected or evolving condition. For example, it is well known that test results for syphilis, hepatitis, or HIV may be negative within the first couple of weeks after exposure, only to turn positive at a later time.

Even if your doctor finds "something" (such as granulomatous spots on your spleen, or evidence in your serum of prior exposure to cytomegalovirus), your doctor may make the judgment that these results would not account for your symptoms and would not be expected to cause harm in the foreseeable future and require no treatment. They are judged to be harmless, self-limited, or leftover signs or scars of previous infections. Thus he will tell you he "found nothing." In other words, sometimes "we found nothing" means that test results fail to indicate there is anything in your body that warrants intervention based on current standards of medical practice. Since many medical problems are self-limited, meaning that they are normally handled by the body without outside help or intervention, most doctors will wisely let nature take its course in those cases. However, such a conclusion is partly a matter of judgment.

Furthermore, even without testing, doctors know that approximately 95 percent of all patients have had exposure to the chicken pox virus and continue to carry the virus in their body without having symptoms. Doctors also know that this hidden virus will cause approximately 20 percent of men and 30 percent of women to develop shingles during their lifetime. However, since prior to the vaccine in 2006 there was no proven treatment for the *Varicella zoster* carrier state, doctors usually waited until the eruption of shingles before undertaking any medical intervention.

Even if nothing abnormal is found or proven, your physician should still have an opinion regarding the likely cause of your concerns or symptoms. You should be informed of that diagnosis even if the doctor believes that your symptoms might be psychosomatic or have an emotional cause. In addition to the diagnosis, you should ask for the results of your tests and keep them in your records for future reference.

Cost-benefit Considerations in Testing

Most likely, you were only tested for conditions that were suspected to be causing your symptoms, and conditions for which there is specific effective treatment available. One of the main reasons why tests for many "nontreatable" conditions are not routinely ordered is because ethical doctors try not to incur unnecessary expenses. Although information obtained from some tests might be interesting, the tests usually won't be ordered if the results are not expected to yield direct benefit in correcting or managing your condition as demonstrated by evidence-based medical practices.

For example, suppose there is a very expensive test that could show whether juvenile-onset diabetes (Type 1 diabetes) was originally triggered by a particular virus. At this time there is no treatment for that virus. Furthermore, if the virus was only the trigger and not an ongoing infection, knowing about the virus would only be of historical or of scientific interest—it would not help reverse or treat the diabetes. If you had no insurance, and if you were charged for such a test, would you feel that this was a worthwhile expenditure? Or would you rather spend your money on treating the existing diabetes? Even if you are insured, should insurance companies pay for tests with no direct current health benefit?

This is partly the reason why we don't always receive full answers to medical questions and why doctors don't test for "everything." In ordering diagnostic tests and interventions, most doctors make a judgment about balancing what it takes to satisfy everyone's curiosity for information against the measurable benefit of treating you successfully. In other words, they make a cost-benefit judgment as well as a risk-benefit judgment. University centers and science laboratories that receive independent funding for research studies and have ethics committees to oversee them can engage in more extended inquiry. In such settings the furthering of science may be considered a higher cause than time and monetary expense. Much of what we know about the biological basis of diseases comes from such settings. However, in a doctor's daily practice, spending the patient's money "unnecessarily" is not considered ethical.

Suppose that after your evaluation, you are told your problem is likely caused by a virus for which there is no specific medical treatment. Which particular virus? As noted above, it isn't helpful to spend money trying to "name that virus" unless it is one of the few treatable ones. Some of the treatable viruses are the various herpesviruses, HIV, hepatitis B and C cytomegalovirus, respiratory syncytial virus, and influenza. For the others, there is currently no treatment other than to allow the body to do its work. To identify the specific nontreatable virus by name would be

what doctors call "academic," in other words, of interest more in acade-
mia than in day-to-day health-care settings. Nevertheless, you should still
ask your physician to give you his or her best educated opinion about
which virus is most likely (for example, could it be cytomegalovirus or
parvovirus B19?), or whether difficult-to-culture bacteria rather than a
virus could be the culprit.

As is clear by now, if you are told nothing was found it still might be
possible that you carry a stealth germ, just not one for which treatment
is available or warranted, or for which the hazards and discomfort and
expense of treatment outweigh the benefit.

Nonetheless, if you were to carry such an infection, it would still be
a good idea to learn about the organism and about possible precautions
against future consequence of the infection, how to protect others, and
to be able to ask your doctor to let you know when effective treatment
becomes available.

You Refuse to Accept the Verdict

Suppose your doctor concludes that you don't have an infectious organism in your system at all. Yet you still don't feel well and are concerned
that the verdict given by your doctor is wrong. What do you do now?

You can raise your particular concerns and ask the doctor to give you
a written answer (using a copy of the worksheet at the end of this book)
about his or her opinion regarding the best diagnostic label that accounts
for your symptoms. Sometimes he or she might say your symptoms are
due to stress or they are psychosomatic (see chapter 6). Other times the
doctor may say "I don't know," and that is fair.

But don't stop there. Ask your doctor whether any of the medications, supplements, or foods you take might contribute to your symptoms. For example, gastrointestinal symptoms such as loose bowels are
often caused by high doses of vitamin C and other supplements or food
intolerances to dairy products or to wheat products. Ask whether you
could minimize or temporarily eliminate any unnecessary medications
such as sleeping medicines, sedatives, antihistamines, high-dose supplements, and so on, which might be causing you to not feel well. Certainly

ask about smoking and using alcohol, if these apply to you. Also ask whether you should take a daily multivitamin with minerals for a few months to correct any minor nutritional deficiencies. If you suspect that you may have some imbalance in your normal bodily flora caused by a prolonged illness or a course of antibiotics, ask whether taking probiotics for a period of time might be helpful (see chapters 2 and 7).

Special Tests

Ask whether certain blood tests have been done that could yield clues to infections or inflammation in your body, such as sedimentation rate, serum protein electrophoresis, and white blood cell count. If you are having ongoing low-grade fevers, was a febrile agglutinins test considered? Or could you have a difficult-to-culture bacterial organism which may require special culture media? If you have had recurrent or persistent infections, ask whether the response of your immune system was tested by measuring quantitative serum immunoglobulin levels (IgG, IgM, IgA) in your blood, or with certain skin tests such as a TB skin test. If these tests were not requested by your doctor, you could ask whether you should have them done; most of these tests are not particularly expensive. If any of these tests are abnormal or suggestive of an infection, then further testing may be considered. However, if they come back normal, then the possibility of a clinically significant infection lessens considerably.

Serum Protein Electrophoresis

A serum protein electrophoresis is a blood test that looks at proteins in the blood called albumin and globulins. Certain patterns of the distribution of these globulins may suggest underlying infection, although they do not definitively prove its presence.

This blood test is most commonly used to check for noninfectious blood disorders such as multiple myeloma. However, if the gamma globulins are broadly elevated ("polyclonal gammopathy" *) it could indicate the presence of certain infections in the body, such as:

Viral infections, especially hepatitis, HIV, mononucleosis, and varicella

Focal or systemic bacterial infections, including endocarditis, osteomyelitis, bacteremia, and possibly tuberculosis

Lung conditions, including chronic bronchitis, bronchiectasis, and pneumonitis

*Polyclonal gammopathy also occurs in the presence of the following noninfectious diseases:

Rheumatologic conditions, including lupus, rheumatoid arthritis, sarcoid, vasculitis

Liver diseases, including cirrhosis, alcoholism, autoimmune hepatitis

Cancers, including lung cancer, ovarian cancer, liver, kidney, and stomach cancers

Blood diseases such as lymphoma, leukemia, thalassemia, and sickle-cell disease

Gastrointestinal conditions such as ulcerative colitis and Crohn's disease

Endocrine conditions including thyroiditis and Graves' disease

Erythrocyte Sedimentation Rate Test

The erythrocyte sedimentation rate (ESR) test is a simple and inexpensive blood test that measures the speed with which red blood cells settle to the bottom of a test tube. Faster-than-normal settling times reflect the presence of inflammatory proteins in the blood, which weigh down the cells.

The ESR test is not specific for infection. However, if elevated, it may be a clue to the possible presence of certain infections. It can be helpful when used as a part of the diagnostic evaluation. If the ESR test is abnormally elevated, further testing may be considered, including a TB skin test, chest X-ray, and serum and urine protein electrophoresis. The ESR test may help detect infection associated with orthopedic implants, children's bacterial infections, and female pelvic infections. It was found to be more accurate in assessing the severity of pelvic infections than a gynecologic examination.

The sedimentation rate may be elevated in various noninfectious inflammatory or destructive processes such as rheumatic conditions, vasculitis, kidney failure, anemia, certain cancers, and even during pregnancy. Also, it can be normal even in the presence of a number of infectious diseases, such as typhoid fever, malaria, or mononucleosis.

Febrile Agglutinins

The febrile agglutinins blood test is used to obtain evidence for the presence of certain infectious diseases, mostly in persons with conditions that cause fever. This test is used most commonly to help diagnose brucellosis, but it is also used to diagnose salmonella, rickettsia, and tularemia infections. It may also be useful in confirming the presence of leukemia and lymphoma.

If you have gastrointestinal symptoms, having a laboratory examination of a sample of your stools should be considered. In addition to a hemoccult test, which checks for traces of blood in the stool and is commonly used to screen for cancer or noncancerous growths in the bowel (done routinely over the age of fifty), a stool parasitology screen (ova and parasites test) can be done. Additionally, a test for *Giardia lamblia* and

Cryptosporidium could be done by various methods. In the case of persons with persistently loose bowels, a test for *Clostridium difficile* toxin, as well as tests for other bacteria, may be ordered. Testing the stool for white blood cells can give a clue to inflammation and possible infection in the bowel. Stool tests are also one way to confirm the active presence of *Helicobacter pylori*.

If a culture of a body surface or body fluid was taken, it is important to ask what culture or testing process was used. A routine "swab" which is taken and sent to the laboratory checks primarily for bacteria or possibly yeast. A culture obtained by this method that comes back negative does not necessarily disprove the presence of a significant virus infection. To isolate particular nonbacterial organisms such as herpes, influenza, certain fungal infections, or even some bacteria, special collection methods, tubes, or plates need to be requested and used by the doctor.

Certain scans may also be considered, such as X-ray, ultrasound, CT (computerized tomography), or MRI (magnetic resonance imaging). To interpret the results, your doctor needs to know what these scans are likely or unlikely to show. Even if infection is present, the scan results might not show anything abnormal, and as such are not fully reliable to detect it (see discussion in chapter 3). The infection must be localized in a cluster large enough to cast a shadow on an X-ray or scan, or have caused some thickening that can be seen on a picture. Sometimes the only clue to an infection is a few "nonspecific" lymph nodes reported on the scan.

Fiber-optic scope tests of the esophagus, stomach, bowels, sinuses, and the pelvic area may be considered to search directly for organisms colonizing the lining of these structures. A simple "look," of course, is also only partly reliable. Even a biopsy or a direct culture is not foolproof.

What other testing is possible? To search more broadly for infections within the body, other types of scans can also be considered. These scans are primarily used to detect the presence of more severe infections, and they may not be very sensitive for picking up inactive or slowly smoldering infections. However, if you suspect an infection and have a persistent discomfort in a well-defined location—let's say the pelvic area, prostate, or sinuses—and CT or MRI scans showed nothing, you could ask your doctor for a white blood cell scan (see sidebar.) The white blood cell scan is not widely known to laypersons since it is usually done in the hospital setting, yet it can have a role in uncovering some hidden infections.

White Blood Cell Scan

A white blood cell scan is used to detect localized infection in various regions of the body, particularly in the abdomen and in bone.

In a white blood cell scan, a blood sample is taken, and the white blood cells, which are the frontline blood cells that fight infection, are labeled with a small amount of radioactive material. The radioactive-labeled white cells are then reinjected into the blood, and imaging is performed on the same day and again the next day by a nuclear medical scanner, during which time the labeled white blood cells have a chance to congregate at the site of infection. Most scans take 30 to 45 minutes.

As the body is scanned, the congregating labeled white cells will "light up" a suspect area. This does not conclusively prove the presence of an infection at that location. Further follow-up tests are needed to prove infection. Falsely abnormal scans can occur where a hematoma or a noninfectious inflammatory condition is present. False negatives may occur in cases of a nonlocalized blood infection such as sepsis, or when the infection is spread diffusely throughout the body, as in hepatitis C or syphilis infection.

Another more sophisticated scan is also available. A PET (positron emission tomography) scan (see sidebar) can sometimes highlight deeply hidden pockets of bacterial or fungal infection in persons who have persistent fever despite antibiotic treatment. This scan is quite expensive, available only at specialty centers, and is therefore seldom used to diagnose infection.

PET (Positron Emission Tomography) Scan

In a PET, or positron emission tomography, scan sugar molecules labeled with a radioactive positron emitter substance (fluorodeoxyglucose) are injected into the bloodstream. The scan locates areas in the body where there is vigorous sugar metabolism, a distinguishing characteristic of infections or tumors. Most commonly this scan is used for detection and documentation of the spread of certain types of cancer.

PET scans are used on rare occasion in patients with fever, who are at high risk for infection, or are significantly ill. It may be useful in identifying clusters of bacterial or fungal infection in patients with blood infections, even when other diagnostic tests are normal.

Even white blood cell scans and PET scans find only infections that are localized to well-defined areas within the body and not those which are spread diffusely throughout the body such as syphilis, hepatitis C, or AIDS. These scans are not foolproof either.

There are other specific blood tests, cultures, skin tests, and serum tests that are used to search for particular organisms such as HIV, Lyme disease, syphilis, *Helicobacter pylori*, tuberculosis, malaria, cytomegalovirus, and the multitude of other germs that afflict human beings. These tests need to be requested individually and specifically by the diagnostician based on suspicion of one or other of these conditions. They are not part of the battery of routine laboratory tests. The number and cost make ordering "one of each" indiscriminately not an option. If such tests are to be considered, you could ask for a consultation with an infectious disease specialist.

Why Not Just Test for "Everything"?

If you don't feel well, you might wonder why your doctor can't just rule out everything using every one of the above tests. As I hope you realize by now, there are no tests that can confirm or rule out every single possibility. Also, for the vast majority of patients, as well as for public health agencies or insurance carriers, the cost of obtaining each and every available test is simply prohibitive. Diagnostic problem solving has to be done by old-fashioned, methodical medical detective work. The mark of a superb diagnostician in any field, whether medicine, science, or engineering, is to obtain the right answer in the minimum necessary number of steps and with the minimum necessary expenditure of time, money, and resources.

As discussed in an earlier chapter, taking a good medical history and careful examination of the patient are critical to the diagnostic process. These steps allow formulation of the working diagnosis, which leads to the consideration and examination of various hypotheses about the cause of the problem at hand and helps determine what further testing is needed, if any.

Most doctors trained in scientific medicine order well-chosen tests to confirm or rule out specific causes for your symptoms. They know which tests are appropriate for which condition or circumstance. They generally avoid so-called fishing expeditions, namely ordering a great number of tests without focus or goal, just to see if anything turns up. Knowledgeable diagnosticians think poorly of those who use such a mindless approach in problem solving.

Empiric Treatment

Despite wisely chosen tests and careful detective work, occasionally there are times when direct proof of a stealth infection cannot be established, even though the doctor might truly suspect one. In such a case, he or she might propose a course of empiric treatment (see Glossary) and prescribe an anti-infective medicine that specifically targets and treats a suspected organism. If a bacterial, fungal, or viral colonization is suspected as an explanation for your symptoms, the doctor will sometimes consider a brief course of an antibacterial, antifungal, or antiviral medication. The medication will be carefully chosen to target the suspected infectious organism(s) in the particular region of the body—pelvis, bowel, stomach, esophagus, sinus, and so on. If it works, such an intervention can provide treatment and at the same time may serve as indirect "proof" of an infection. CAUTION: Consider such treatment only under the supervision of your physician, and only if you are not allergic to such medicines.

For certain skin conditions that are suspected to be due to infection, the doctor might suggest a trial of some simple topical remedies. For example, a small patch of the skin affected by a suspected infection may be treated with povidone-iodine (Betadine) solution, a water-washable antiseptic solution that kills bacteria, fungi, and viruses. It is the same solution that is used by health professionals in the hospital to decontaminate their own skin as well as the skin of patients prior to surgery. This solution should be used with caution, because some persons are allergic to iodine, and povidone-iodine could also make certain noninfectious conditions worse. It should not be used in open wounds. However, if the patch of abnormal skin treated with povidone-iodine begins to normalize, you may conclude that an infectious agent was part of the culprit, and this may be useful information for you and your doctor. CAUTION: Consider such trials only under the direction of your doctor, and only if you know you are not allergic to iodine. This iodine-containing solution is not to be put in or near your eyes or up your nose or come in contact with your mouth or other mucous membranes. It should not be swallowed or taken internally. Also, except for a brief rinse, open wounds should generally not be treated with providone-iodine because repeated use inhibits granulation tissue formation, which is what is needed for wounds to heal.

In all cases empiric treatment should be done only under your doctor's close supervision, since all medications, whether prescription or nonprescription, have potential adverse effects, including severe allergies. Many doctors are understandably reluctant to treat empirically with antibiotics or antimicrobials because of concerns about overuse of these medicines and possible adverse effects, especially if they don't have proof of a diagnosis. Nevertheless, sometimes such treatment is less invasive, less expensive, and safer than scope tests, biopsies, or exploratory surgery. Underuse of judicious empiric treatment is as much of a mistake as overuse.

If your symptoms improve and promptly resolve after such treatment, then it can be surmised that an infection was a likely cause of your problem. At times a clue to hidden stealth infection may arise when some of your problems or symptoms disappear while an unrelated infection is treated, for example, pelvic or prostate symptoms improve after antibiotic treatment for sinus infection. Another interesting clue to hidden infections I have seen was improvement of certain unexplained symptoms after receiving a shot of gamma globulin (a temporary immune booster against common infections) given as protection against Hepatits A exposure.

Suppose you were treated with an empiric course of an anti-infective or antibiotic and your symptoms cleared. Ask your doctor for an opinion about what infection they thought you actually had. This information is useful to protect yourself against a relapse or recurrence. Also ask whether you might have passed the presumed infection on to someone else, such as a sex partner.

Getting Another Opinion

If you have taken all the steps outlined above and you do not have a satisfactory explanation for your ongoing symptoms, or if your doctor doesn't feel comfortable ordering further tests or treating you empirically, what should you do? You could ask for a second opinion, or an opinion from an infectious disease specialist. Even if insurance doesn't pay for the extra consultation, it may be worth paying a consultant's fee out of pocket. Further testing recommended by the consultant could be discussed with your primary physician.

What if there is still no proof of an infection? If you have already seen your doctor, obtained a second opinion, and received a thorough examination and testing by a consultant such as an infectious disease expert, and there is still no finding of an infection, then it is quite unlikely that you have a significant stealth infection underlying your symptoms or which threatens your health. At this point, some will *still* not be satisfied with the answer and wonder if a hidden infection is possible. The general answer is, almost anything is possible, and cautious doctors never say never. Diagnostic answers are almost never foolproof. Most thoughtful physicians will advise you whether a suspected condition may be quite likely, somewhat likely, unlikely, or extremely unlikely (see worksheet at the end of the book). In medicine, that is often the best answer we can give. You could still be an asymptomatic carrier of hidden organisms such as the *Varicella zoster* virus that could give you shingles at some time in the future. However, this is also the time to seriously consider and accept other noninfectious explanations for your problems.

At such a point the best you can do is to allow some time to pass. Certain infections may resolve or continue to evolve or emerge with time. As time passes, be aware of events that may affect your symptoms. If you take antibiotics for some other reason, such as dental work or a bronchial infection, note whether there is improvement of your other symptoms while you are on these antibiotics. Such improvement could be an important and useful clue. Always report such observations to your doctor.

In the event that you continue to have evolving, persistent, or new symptoms, return to your doctor periodically for checkups to see whether new clues have emerged. At such a visit, a new set of blood or urine tests may be done, and some tests that were originally negative might turn positive or yield new findings.

Do not give up on your doctor. Return for a recheck and bring even better organized information so he or she can gain a better perspective of your problem. In a complicated case, a diagnostician doesn't always see the whole picture of a partially assembled puzzle on the first try. If allowed to look at and think about the puzzle a few times, especially after taking a breather, he or she may ultimately get the picture. The same consideration applies to a specialist. When a specialist sees you and examines you one single time, he or she may give you an initial take on what they believe they see. If you still don't have a satisfactory diagnosis, giving them a second chance to reconsider their assessment can be useful. Reconsidering a diagnosis by retaking a history and redoing the examination is often the best way to uncover a complicated, hidden, and hard-to-find infection or other medical condition.

There Are Diseases Other Than Stealth Infections

Though the subject of this book is stealth infections, you should not become obsessed with the possibility of having a lurking stealth infection, to the exclusion of other explanations for your symptoms. Most of the various medical conditions and diseases described in medical textbooks can cause a person to not feel well. Endocrine conditions such as underactive or overactive thyroid, underactive or overactive adrenals, diabetes, or anemia can cause you to feel poorly. Cancer, tumors, and other serious problems should also be kept in mind. Finally, diet and other habits should be taken into account. All such conditions need to be considered in evaluating someone who doesn't feel right before trying to pin the blame on a stealth infection. In fact, many screening tests ordered as part of a standard blood panel are designed to uncover these other underlying abnormalities.

However, suppose that none of these other evaluations turn up anything, either. Could it be something like candida or toxic mold? Or could it all be "in your head"?

Molds in Your Home and Candida: Germs Unlikely to Make You Sick

With all your tests coming out negative, friends might suggest that your symptoms are due to something much more obvious than a stealth germ: either toxic molds in your home, or candida in your body. Some persons believe that these conditions are easily overlooked by doctors and that traditional medicine underestimates their damaging effects. Is that really true?

There are occasional circumstances when certain health problems can be caused by household mold and candida. The controversy involves establishing a cause-and-effect relationship between these organisms and a variety of symptoms, such as chronic fatigue, malaise, mood swings, palpitations, irritable bowels, irritated skin and eyes, and an irritated windpipe. Remember, correlation does not mean causation. Overestimating a causal relationship is just as much of a mistake as underestimating it. Also, one should be cautious when attributing all symptoms to a single cause rather than multiple causes.

We need to be careful not to convict an innocent bystander, even if they look suspicious, when a crime has been committed (as we already saw with *Haemophilus influenzae* bacteria, which is a latecomer and bystander in some cases of viral influenza). The presence of a germ at the scene of an illness does not prove that it is the direct cause of someone's symptoms or medical problems. Keep in mind the dramatic physical reaction of persons who faint when someone is about to draw blood from them (usually jokingly described as an allergy to needles), which is a common example of a conditioned response to a specific stimulus. Other examples of true physical symptoms caused by a conditioned response of the brain are "butterflies" in the stomach that some persons feel when asked to perform in front of others, actual vomiting when seeing a sickening sight, crushing chest pressure when receiving sudden devastating news, or getting real goosebumps when hearing about something exciting. Hence the caution about attributing symptoms to contact with a biological substance, when it may be a conditional response.

Cultures taken from damp buildings suspected of being the source of toxic mold diseases not only grow molds, but also grow a large number of other organisms, including gram-negative bacteria and mycobacteria. Yet these other organisms are not generally blamed for causing symptoms or problems by advocates of the mold–illness connection.

Toxic Buildings and Toxic Molds

In the case of molds in damp buildings, the concern is often not about direct infection or even illness caused by the live spores of the molds in the manner of a stealth germ, but rather exposure to the toxins the molds produce.

In considering potential reactions of persons exposed to or residing in moldy buildings, such reactions are classified into at least six categories: irritant effects, nonspecific respiratory symptoms, allergic sensitization, reaction to fungal toxins, psychogenic reactions, and infection. Indoor mold exposures generally do not cause true fungal infections in persons with normal immune systems. In fact, true infections caused by fungal spores are primarily acquired outdoors.

Symptoms of irritation could be due to toxic organic chemicals shed by the fungus, which can produce irritation of the eyes, nose, and windpipe. However, such symptoms are usually time limited and occur when the person is in close proximity to the fungus shedding toxin, and will improve when the person leaves the area. Children in damp indoor environments are more likely than others to have respiratory problems, but it is not clear whether the culprit is fungus or some other factor. It also appears to be true that persons who are particularly susceptible to allergies can develop significant allergic sensitization from mold-toxin exposure, which can cause asthma, hypersensitivity pneumonitis, or allergic sinusitis.

There are some rather severe human illnesses (poisonings) related to heavy exposure to the toxins produced by molds, among them ergotism (caused by toxins from *Aspergillus* species), alimentary-toxic aleukia (caused by toxins of *Fusarium*), liver disease (caused by toxins of aspergillus), and other conditions. Animals that ingest large amounts of toxins produced by molds in their feed can also develop severe problems. However, in human beings and animals, ingestion of large amounts of toxin-carrying substances, or heavy, persistent contact with the toxin, such as lying on contaminated straw, is usually required before symptoms of poisoning occur. These symptoms may include a significant skin rash or gastrointestinal symptoms. With rare exception, in situations where less direct contact occurs, such as students attending classes in a damp school building, the cause-and-effect relationship between damp buildings and a multitude of various reported symptoms is less clear.

As already noted, conditions attributed to indoor exposure to toxic molds in damp buildings generally are not caused by the molds growing as stealth germs in your body. If there is a problem, it is usually not the fungus itself but the toxin that is believed to be the cause, and as such, treatment with antimicrobials is not warranted. Molds may act as stealth germs in your house, or as stealth germs in a building or even the hospital, but that would be the subject of a different book.

Common Human Fungal Infections

What about other fungal infections, particularly candida? If some fluid from your body is cultured and candida grows in the culture, should you receive prompt treatment for the proven infection? Or should candida be considered normal flora?

Most physicians and biologists accept that various fungi in small numbers are part of the human body's normal flora and that otherwise healthy persons are quite resistant to being internally and invasively overrun by most fungi and molds, including candida.

There are certain well-known conditions where fungal organisms that are not part of the normal flora invade the body. Mostly these are familiar skin and body-surface problems such as athlete's foot, jock itch, *Tinea versicolor*, and others. These fungi cause the well-known redness, itching, and sometimes scaling or oozing of the affected skin or other surfaces. As a rule, such infections do not make a person feel ill or experience fatigue. Even severe fungal infestation of the toenails does not cause malaise and does not spread into the blood or the body's interior.

A lesser-known "invasive" fungal infection of the body surface and lymph nodes is sporotrichosis, which is caused by the fungus *Sporothrix schenckii*. It may become inoculated under the skin and spread to the lymph nodes in persons handling certain plants, such as fungus-contaminated rosebushes. Diagnosis and treatment for such fungal infestations is available.

Candida

Monilia (*Candida albicans*), a member of the normal flora of the body, can cause health problems under certain circumstances. It is the cause of most "yeast infections," which we have already discussed. It is extremely rare for it to spread in the form of disseminated candidiasis to the true internal organs of the body—liver, spleen, kidney, or inside of the eyeball—nor does it circulate in the bloodstream in otherwise healthy individuals. One special group where this may occur is intravenous drug abusers. Those with candida circulating in their blood usually have very significant immune problems and become severely ill. Evaluation and management of these patients is beyond the scope of this book.

There must be a significant excess overgrowth of candida in order for it to cause symptoms. Unfortunately there is no specific number of colonies that can be used as criteria for the "excess." Most often such overgrowth occurs on skin or mucous membranes and is obvious to the naked eye. However, some of these surfaces are inside the body, such as the lining of the esophagus, the throat, or sinuses, and therefore the yeast infection may not be directly visible. In those instances candida can mimic a stealth germ.

Candida infection is occasionally overlooked in the esophagus (*Candida esophagitis*). The esophagus or throat may become colonized by candida organisms in someone who is now or was recently undergoing treatment with antibiotics or prednisone, or in someone who uses corticosteroid inhalers for asthma. The affected patient usually feels a persistent burning sensation in their esophagus or throat, which is not relieved by antacids or nonprescription lozenges.

Since these surfaces are not readily visible from the outside, the candida infestation may not be considered, unless the throat or esophagus is examined with a scope. Even health-care professionals often attribute the symptoms to simple acid reflux. If you have such burning of the esophagus and you fit the above criteria, you should ask your doctor whether candida might be a factor. Empiric treatment with an antiyeast preparation to see if the symptoms will clear is usually a simple measure, and may be curative. A scope examination of the throat or esophagus could prove candida infestation, but may also find other unexpected findings, such as an eruption of herpes or canker sores, which may cause similar burning or discomfort not relieved by antacids.

There is little or no evidence that in an absence of any other findings chronic fatigue syndrome or chronic aches and pains are due to candida. As a rule, someone who doesn't feel well and has had extensive normal laboratory tests, does not abuse intravenous drugs, and does not have severe immune deficiency problems is highly unlikely to be the victim of stealth molds or stealth candida in the body.

The Fungal Infections You May Not Think Of

Those who are focused primarily on candida and toxic molds sometimes overlook the fact that there are several well-described medical conditions caused by other fungal organisms. From the stealth germ perspective, infection caused by certain outdoor fungi may be of greater potential interest. Spores of such organisms can remain in the body as stealth germs, with the possibility of re-emerging from within when the body's immune system becomes suppressed.

The conditions histoplasmosis, blastomycosis, coccidioidomycosis (known as "valley fever" in California), and cryptococcosis are caused by fungal organisms whose spores are inhaled by otherwise healthy persons with normal immune systems. Evidence of prior exposure to these microbes is sometimes found as small spots (granulomas) on X-rays of the lungs or the spleen or other internal organs taken for an unrelated reason. A person with such test results sometimes recalls having had a "really bad" respiratory infection, which eventually cleared up. Often such persons have no recollection of ever being ill. Interestingly, an outbreak of valley fever occurred after the 1994 earthquake in the Los Angeles area, when dirt containing the spores was shaken off the nearby mountains, causing an unusually large number of cases of coccidioidomycosis infections and exposures.

Generally these fungi cause only transient respiratory infections in otherwise healthy individuals. A few persons became more seriously ill. In fighting off the exposure, the immune system has a unique response, called a "granulomatous reaction," which walls away the spores in the lymph nodes, the lungs, or the spleen.* Though trapped in the granulomas, some of the spores remain alive, though dormant. In this way, these organisms can take up residence as stealth germs in the body, though after doing so they generally do not cause any symptoms or ongoing problems.

---

* The body's immune system responds to exposure to fungal spores by a different mechanism than it responds to viruses or bacteria. It is the cellular part of the immune system that responds (activated lymphocytes), in contrast to the chemical immune response (immune globulins), which goes into action when bacterial and viral infections attack.

However, under the right circumstances, these fungal organisms can become reactivated and start an infection that arises from within. In persons receiving chemotherapy or medicines that suppress the immune system, or sometimes even during pregnancy, these organisms can suddenly reemerge from their hiding place behind the walled-off granulomas and begin to cause fever, lung symptoms, or other signs of illness. Otherwise, they will continue to lurk in the body, waiting for an opportunity to take advantage of the host when his or her defenses are down. Preventive treatment is generally not recommended for asymptomatic carriers of these fungal organisms, as the risk outweighs the benefit. The only granulomatous disease for which preventive treatment of asymptomatic individuals is recommended is tuberculosis, a non-fungal infection.

There is another rare but potentially severe fungal condition that may infect persons with significant respiratory problems such as asthma, emphysema, or other severe lung disease. This is allergic pulmonary aspergillosis, caused by the fungus *Aspergillus fumigatus*. However, the mere presence of this fungus in sputum does not prove that the person's asthma is caused by this fungus. Often this fungus is only an innocent bystander.

When pulmonary aspergillosis makes you sick, it causes an obvious illness, not a stealthy one. Invasion of the respiratory tract by this organism causes severe asthmalike breathing problems, including shortness of breath and wheezing. It may also cause a severe sinus infection.

Both immunocompetent and immunocompromised patients can have a lung infection that is caused by the spores of other fungal conditions such as cryptococcosis, an infection that may spread to internal organs. Infection with other fungal disease-causing organisms, such as *Pneumocystis*, the rare pigmented fungi *Fusarium*, and Zygomycetes, occurs almost exclusively in patients who have severe immune deficiencies. These infections generally progress rapidly with obvious and severe symptoms, and their management is outside the scope of this book.

If there is concern about such fungal infections or exposure to fungal organisms, and if simple answers are not forthcoming, you should consult an infectious disease specialist, who will be able to put X-ray, laboratory test results, and other findings into proper perspective. Remember that mere presence of a germ on the body or on a culture plate does not prove that the germ is the cause of one's symptoms or problems. It is a time-honored medical maxim that one should treat the patient and not the laboratory test results. It is the role of the diagnostician to use wisdom as well as knowledge in evaluating information that may appear contradictory, counterintuitive, and confusing to a layperson, and then advise the patient regarding the meaning of the results and the best course of action.

If you have been evaluated and are advised that your symptoms are not caused by toxic molds, candida, or other fungal organisms, and your tests show no indications of other infections or other diseases, could it be all in your head? The next section addresses that issue.

Could It Be in Your Head?

If all evidence for infection or disease keeps turning up negative, one eventually needs to raise the question about the role of the "head," or more accurately the brain, in explaining why you may not feel right. We all know that the brain largely determines how and what we feel. That is why under anesthesia, when the brain is "disconnected," a person doesn't feel one way or another, nor feel anything at all for that matter, despite the continued presence of diseases or cutting by the surgeon's knife. The brain also can cause us to feel instantly devastated by bad news or elated with good news. The brain can also cause us to faint when we see something frightening, or cause us to get sick to our stomach when we see something nauseating.

Major structural malfunctions of the brain, such as a brain tumor, fluid on the brain, a stroke, or an injured area are readily detected, since they appear on brain scans as abnormal areas. However, there is no simple test for microscopic or chemical malfunctions in the brain. For example, ordinary brain scans of a person during a severe and incapacitating migraine headache show no visible or discernable abnormalities.

Blood samples can be readily used for measuring hormone levels and other abnormalities or deficiencies in the body and the blood. However, chemicals in the brain cannot easily be measured, in part because of the so-called blood-brain barrier (see Glossary). This microfilter of capillaries in the head prevents many substances from leaking out of the brain into the blood, as well as preventing transfer of many chemicals from the blood into the brain. Therefore, chemicals produced by the brain are usually not present in the bloodstream but are retained in the brain fluid or brain cells. Deficiencies of such brain chemicals can be proven only by sampling the brain tissues, a procedure that is almost never done for obvious reasons.

Many neurotransmitters are at work in the brain. Some of these are acetylcholine, noradrenalin, serotonin, gamma-aminobutyric acid (GABA), glutamate, dopamine, and corticotropin-releasing factor. Deficiency or overactivity of any of these chemicals is possible. Additionally, the brain is an extremely complex "macrochip" with mind-bogglingly intricate connections among nerve cells. The "wiring" may develop microscopic glitches, malformations, or short-circuits, which are too small to show up on CT, MRI, or other brain scans, even though they may cause significant alterations in how one feels and how the brain operates.

The Brain and How We Feel

A commonly given illustration of how a perfectly normal brain can profoundly influence how one feels is as follows: A completely healthy man is down on his luck. He is financially broke. His family has deserted him, he has no friends, and winds up homeless on the street. He feels weary, dejected, depressed, has aches and pains, and generally feels miserable. He buys a lottery ticket. The next day he checks the numbers on his ticket against the winning numbers and finds a perfect match! In one instant, without anything else having happened, just by seeing six little marks on a small slip of paper, this person changes from feeling terrible to feeling marvelous and elated.

Can the brain in one instant really produce such change in how a person feels? How can this happen without taking anything, or without appreciable time for the brain to manufacture new or more chemicals? Can the brain's perception of how a person feels be changed in an instant, as if a light switch were thrown? Clearly it happens. No question that, independent from the rest of the body, the brain has a major role in determining how we feel minute to minute and day to day, both physically and emotionally.

Human brains are not all identical. There are many inherited or inborn differences and variations that significantly influence how our brain makes us feel. One discovery involving stealth germs is that some of them may do hit-and-run damage to the intricate neurochemical circuitry of the developing brain. Schizophrenia, seizure disorders, and mental retardation are potentially linked to exposure of the brain to certain infections. Such exposure may occur while in the mother's womb or during infancy or early childhood. Damage from such an infection can predispose a person to have minimal, mild, moderate, or perhaps severe brain problems later on in life.

Those with a mild case may not even realize that some minor malfunction in their brain is causing them to not feel right. As such, they may continue a quest to find some other factor in the body outside of the brain that explains how they feel. They may be reading this book to see if the active presence of a stealth infection could be the culprit. Obviously, there are many other conditions besides infections that can affect the brain during development or childhood, including chemicals, physical injuries, as well as certain inheritable deficiencies. Any combination of these factors can give rise to conditions such as bipolar disorder, seizure disorders, attention deficit disorders, and other conditions.

Rather than stealth infections, many persons who do not feel well in fact have minor flaws in their brain's wiring, or deficiencies or overproduction of the chemicals produced in their brain. Unfortunately, these brain defects or deficiencies are largely impossible to measure at this time with commonly used tests, and their existence must be surmised by the examiner based on his or her knowledge of these conditions. Even a severe brain problem such as Parkinson's disease shows no abnormality on conventional scans or other laboratory tests. Parkinson's disease is fully verifiable only after the patient dies, and even then only if specific pathologic examinations are ordered.

Variations in the Normal Brain

The effect of external factors on the day-to-day workings of the brain also varies significantly among different individuals. An interesting example of how the response of the neurochemistry and neurocircuitry of the brain varies can be seen by the differing effects of alcohol on various normal healthy persons. If a group of persons ingests alcohol-containing drinks with identical ingredients and identical alcohol content, what result will be observed? Some will become drowsy and sleepy. Others will not be drowsy at all, and in fact some may feel pleasantly relaxed. Some will become annoying and argumentative after drinking. Sadly, a rare individual will lose self-control, becoming belligerent and challenging, or will run into problems by using poor judgment. A few become incorrigible alcoholics. These are all responses of the normal human brain to an identical ingested chemical substance. Such varied results are also observed in response to other substances, possibly also to infectious stimuli. Brain scans of the individuals exhibiting such varied responses show no simple detectable variations or abnormalities. How can this be?

Different persons evidently have different neurochemistries or different circuit patterns in their brains that account for such contradictory reactions in how a person feels when exposed to the same environment, same substance, the same stimuli, or even the same medical condition. This may be part of the reason why some persons feel well and others don't feel well under identical circumstances. Unfortunately there is no simple way yet to differentiate the specific brain patterns that predict individual responses. In the future there will likely be such tests, and there are some available in hospitals and research centers.

Is Your Problem Psychosomatic?

Ultimately, if you do not have any detectable medical abnormalities in your body, and the conclusion is that your symptoms originate "in your head," should you interpret that to mean that you have a problem of character, a psychosomatic illness, or even a personality problem? Possibly, but not necessarily.

Unfortunately terms used in everyday public conversation are still cluttered with labels left over from prior years and centuries. Some of these have questionable, misleading, prejudicial and biased meanings and origins. Take for example "hysteria," originally meaning "wandering uterus," or "cretin," meaning mentally retarded from congenital hypothyroidism, or "hyper," from hyperthyroidism. There's also "demented," from the Latin *"demens"* literally meaning "away from one's mind." Labeling everything for which there is no easily demonstrable physical cause as "psychosomatic" is an archaic generalization. Such terms are used by laypersons, but hopefully not by medical scientists, who generally try to use terms that more specifically describe or classify symptoms. Prejudicial generalizations should be avoided, and diagnoses should be based on the modern understanding of biology, biochemistry, and neurochemistry of the brain.

But does that mean that there aren't psychological causes for some physical symptoms? It is true that when some healthy persons are under stress—or more accurately, "distressed"—they may not feel well, and may seek attention for their situational distress by highlighting physical symptoms. However, it is not true that the brain of every healthy-appearing adult is wired perfectly/uniformly/normally and produces entirely ideal/perfect/normal amounts of neurochemicals and responses at all times. One cannot reduce to simplistic terms the extremely complicated fields of neurophysiology, neurochemistry, and neuroendocrinology. How some physically healthy–appearing persons feel is not entirely an issue of their character or their circumstance.

We can usually recognize otherwise normal persons who are distressed, grieving, inappropriately elated, or delirious. However, in absence of these causes a person may still have a feeling of malaise arising from the brain. In that case, a way to describe this malaise is to say that they have a neurophysiologic, neurobehavioral, or neuropsychiatric problem. It could even be characterized as a neurochemical circuitry dysfunction of the brain. More precise classifications are attempted in neurology or psychiatry textbooks. Such disorders of the brain, whether inborn or acquired, certainly exist, despite the opinion of certain groups or individuals to the contrary. As time goes on, we will be able to prove that many persons whose primary symptom is ongoing malaise may have true defects in their brain's neurochemistry and neurocircuitry.

Some remedies already exist or are being developed for these deficiencies. Medicines such as antidepressants, psychostimulants, and sedatives are somewhat poorly targeted remedies. Nevertheless, in certain individuals they can produce excellent results. Empiric treatment applies not only to stealth germs but can also apply to neuropsychiatric problems.

If, after a thorough medical checkup, you suspect that part of your malaise may be coming from your head/brain, you should consider evaluation by a neurologist, counselor, or psychiatrist, or talk to your doctor about medications that might help your central nervous system. Use of such medications is no more a sign of weakness of character than using a thyroid supplement to treat an underactive thyroid condition.

There are other things you can do to help yourself feel better. You can regulate or stabilize your sleep cycle if it is irregular. Eliminate excess alcohol, tobacco, sedatives, and stimulants and consider taking multivitamins. Engage in healthy activities such as exercise and practice relaxation techniques. During the winter consider lighting rooms more brightly during the daytime to counteract the gloom. At night make your bedroom quiet and dark when you try to sleep. Then ask your doctor to treat any symptoms that remain.

In the meantime, listen to your body. Keep alert for possible evolving medical problems. Even a person who has "something in their head," and is high-strung or depressed, can develop other illnesses, too. Be sure that your treating physician does not fail to consider and reconsider the possibility that you may have two or more different problems at the same time: a "nervous" disorder as well as other evolving conditions, such as a smoldering stealth germ.

7. Treatment Expectations

To Treat or Not to Treat

After all is said and done, suppose you find out that you do indeed have an infectious organism lurking in your body. You are ready to rid yourself of it, only to find out that there is no treatment for your infection. Suppose you carry a herpesvirus. Why can't we just get rid of all herpesviruses from our system, including herpes simplex 1 and 2, herpesvirus 8, *Varicella zoster*, and cytomegalovirus? Finding hepatitis C in your system may also lead to such questions: Isn't it harmful to leave this organism circulating in your system? Doesn't it increase your risk of cancer of the liver? There are some known treatments for it. Let's use them, treat the invader, and be done with it.

Not So Fast

Treatment of medical conditions, including infections, is tempered by the simple fact that medical interventions are almost never totally harmless. Furthermore, some conditions respond readily to treatment while others may not. Some treatments are potentially toxic, others not. There may not be medicines or treatments available for certain organisms. As we already noted, there are numerous medicines available to fight bacteria and several medicines against fungi, but there are few antiviral medicines. Even medicines that have been proven effective against the herpesviruses are suppressive, not curative.

Undertaking treatment is not based on simple common sense. In deciding to treat, the physician who practices evidence-based medicine usually turns to outcome studies. He or she does not initiate treatment simply because a germ is present. Remember, we have to treat the patient, not the finding. The doctor needs to determine whether the patient will benefit from the intervention and whether potential toxicity is outweighed by the potential benefit of the treatment. *Primum non nocere*: first, do no harm.

How can we determine such benefit? When treatments for particular conditions first become available, groups of persons are treated and followed to see what results the treatment produces, and such results are eventually compiled in the medical literature. Although there are numerous outcome studies for conditions such as cancer, few studies of the long-term benefits of treating or not treating stealth germs have been documented. Furthermore, there are very few valid long-term outcome studies with nonprescription or natural remedies.

Even with the reported studies, we must keep in mind that not all clinical trials are equally reliable. Even if a preliminary study or small survey shows that certain treatments provide dramatic benefits, the results may not be confirmed when repeated with a larger number of patients or replicated by other researchers who adhere to more rigorous scientific criteria. Sometimes recommendations that initially appear in the medical literature are later overturned when additional experiments fail to confirm the original result. Additionally, one cannot generalize the results of a study done with middle-aged persons to persons who are in their nineties, for example. Over time, these are the sources of apparently contradictory and confusing recommendations.

We need to look to qualified persons to interpret and put in perspective the entire body of information available on a particular treatment, rather than relying on the claims of one particular study, a mistake commonly made by the popular press and by laypersons. One way to get a critical perspective of these smaller studies is to read the editorial commentary in peer-reviewed medical textbooks or journals. You can find these journals in any medical center's library, numerous public libraries, and many of these studies are available online.

Bright persons often try to draw their own conclusions about medical matters by the use of logic. But outcomes of medical interventions and treatments cannot be predicted by logic alone—one needs to know the results of actual studies. Those who study medical thinking repeatedly conclude that to make wise treatment decisions and diagnoses, one needs to have content knowledge, not just a logical mind (though the latter is definitely necessary, too).

Keep in mind also that most medical studies are not designed to yield a global pronouncement on the matter under consideration. They are designed to give limited answers to specific questions as they pertain to the limited group of individuals who were part of the study. In the case of infections, we need to be cautious when deciding that a particular study result can be applied as a general rule to all such infections, and that the same conclusions are appropriate for all forms and severities of that infection. The results of a focused study won't reliably predict how such infections may behave in certain individuals with their own peculiarities or other coexisting conditions. Hence we always need to look at a patient's specific case and decide whether the result of a particular study even pertains to him or her. This is why the use of computerized decision-making tools may be problematic in making treatment decisions, unless the programming becomes sophisticated enough to account for all individual variations. In real life, some persons need to be treated one way, and others require a different approach.

Chlamydia and Heart Disease

An example of the complexities of treatment decisions concerns *Chlamydia pneumoniae* in the case of atherosclerosis. The presence of *C. pneumoniae* in humans appears to be associated with an increased likelihood of atherosclerosis and heart attack. In a recent limited study over two years, 162 patients who had a recent heart attack were treated with an antibiotic to help eradicate chlamydia from their systems. Those who intermittently took a particular antibiotic in an attempt to clear chlamydia were found not to have a lower risk of near-term recurrent heart attacks.

The press reported this, and some doctors accepted it as evidence that treatment of chlamydia with antibiotics in persons with heart disease doesn't work. But, what do they mean by heart disease, and what do they mean when they say it doesn't work? What do they mean by "antibi-otics"? Should we apply this conclusion to everyone with any type of heart disease or even to those who have not yet developed symptomatic heart disease but are merely at risk? Does the conclusion of this study also apply to all patients at all ages, whether you have had heart surgery or not? Do these results apply whether you were treated for two years, five years, or ten years? Is it equally applicable to patients who may or may not have evidence in their blood tests of low-grade infection or exposure to the chlamydia organism? Do these results apply to any and all antimi-crobials? Of course not.

We all long for simple rules to follow to keep ourselves healthy, and individuals as well as persons in the media attempt to distill the results of medical studies into such simple rules. However, one needs to be very cautious in making general pronouncements from the results of such studies. The press release in the above case was entitled "Antibiotics do not prevent heart attacks." Such a statement is not only inaccurate but also misleading. For example, the study in question was not done with a variety of antibiotics or antimicrobials, only one, gatifloxacin. A more accurate headline would have been, "One particular antibiotic does not reduce the chance of recurrent heart attacks over a two-year period in a small number of patients."

This study did not treat persons who have never had a heart attack to see if antibiotic treatment would help them avoid a heart attack in the first place. No conclusion whatsoever can be made from this study about whether antibiotics in general reduce the chance of a first heart attack. The study did not sort out persons with congestive heart failure or heart valve problems, and there was no extended follow-up of patients for five, ten, or twenty years, only for a period of two years. As a result, we do not know whether such treatment might have reduced the chance of devel-oping other circulatory problems or a stroke years later. We only know that for those who had already had a heart attack previously, a certain short-term outcome was not altered by one certain medicine. We there-fore cannot yet make any general conclusions about chlamydia and "heart conditions." Seek the recommendation of specialists with a perspective.

Simply reading newspaper or Internet summaries or headlines may be misleading and detrimental.

Treating the Ulcer Bacteria

Interestingly, under certain circumstances physicians are reluctant to treat patients with the ulcer bacteria *H. pylori*. Short-term outcome studies have shown that persons harboring the organism whose only symptom of is acid indigestion do not notice much improvement in their acid indigestion symptoms after antibiotic treatment. Given the concern that the organism may develop resistance to antimicrobials if antibiotics are overused, some physicians do not prescribe medication unless the patient has active stomach ulcers.

Leaving *H. pylori* untreated, however, raises an important question: Regardless of symptoms, isn't there a risk in leaving an infection smoldering in the stomach for decades? The current belief is that chronic inflammation caused by the organism may be a predisposing factor in the development of stomach cancer. Will a person be better off twenty years from now if they were treated or not treated? Such study results do not exist at this time. Such studies would require too much time—patients are lost to follow-up and persons coordinating the study retire or lose interest. There are also significant ethical issues with withholding potential treatment over extended periods of time. Since they are too cumbersome and expensive to design and implement, such studies are almost never done. As a result, physicians must still use their best judgment in making such treatment decisions and rely upon consensus recommendations from experts who have a broad perspective on the subject.

Treating Hepatitis C

In the case of hepatitis C, treatment decisions are even more complicated. In considering treatment, one needs to balance the potential toxicity of treatment against the expected virulence of the organism when left untreated. Currently available treatments for hepatitis C carrier state are rather toxic in the short term. Some persons may in fact be left untreated based on risk-versus-benefit considerations, despite concerns about the long-term consequences of the infection. A good question to be raised is: Does eradication of the infection significantly reduce the likelihood of future liver cancer? Or once you have had the infection, are you still at risk?

A Couple of Notorious Conditions—Should They Be Treated Empirically with Antimicrobials?

There are two notable conditions where the possibility of an infectious cause has been raised, though not proven. These conditions are chronic fatigue syndrome (CFS) and Gulf War syndrome. Stealth germs have been suspected by some health care professionals and also by patients to cause these conditions, even if not in all, but perhaps in some of the sufferers. Are there outcome studies to show that these conditions might benefit from empiric treatment for presumed infection?

Chronic Fatigue Syndrome

Suspicions have been raised over the years that CFS may be an infectious or a post-infectious condition. What is CFS? According to medical textbooks, CFS is defined as at least six months of new-onset symptoms of fatigue accompanied by infectious, rheumatological, and neuropsychiatric symptoms that cannot be attributed to or explained by other known medical conditions or diagnoses. However, it has been noted that Lyme disease, a treatable bacterial infection, is known to produce a constellation of symptoms similar to CFS.

The reason that the possibility of an infectious trigger for CFS has been raised is because of the existence of conditions such as Lyme disease and because CFS sometimes starts and evolves suddenly after an influenza-like onset, especially during the winter months. A postviral syndrome that produces symptoms similar to CFS is not uncommon following severe viral infections. However, persistence of known infectious agents in persons with the above-defined diagnosis of CFS has not been reliably demonstrated. One possible explanation is that an infection may indeed trigger CFS, but that sustained activation and reaction of the immune system, not a persistent active infection, causes the chronic malaise or fatigue.

Over the years, there has been scattered evidence that certain infectious agents, such as cytomegalovirus, Q fever, Epstein-Barr virus, and viral meningitis, can cause symptoms of chronic fatigue. However, the actual presence of these organisms in the body could not be proven. It is now believed that those with chronic fatigue syndrome may be suffering a final result of various causes—some infectious, some not. Some likely have immune reactions to previous infections. Most are unlikely to have active ongoing infections that would benefit from treatment. This partly explains why no single treatment has been shown to be effective in all cases of CFS.

Nevertheless, consultation with an infectious disease specialist is generally considered worthwhile for patients who have symptoms of chronic fatigue and malaise in order to find the occasional case of a treatable hidden stealth infection. Abnormalities on diagnostic tests outlined in chapter 6 could be a clue to an underlying infection. As usual, one should be cautious about applying blanket labels to persons who do not feel well, or generalizing the results of treatment in one group of persons to all others with similar symptoms.

Over the years, there have been attempts to administer empiric treatment with antibacterials, antivirals, and even immune globulin to groups of individuals with CFS, just in case there was a hidden infectious cause. With some exceptions, the results have been generally disappointing, and therefore empiric treatment with antimicrobials is usually not done. Even for those whose CFS is found to be related to infection with the Lyme disease organism, treatment with antibiotics appears to be after the fact and often does not help the patient feel better even when the organisms are eradicated. This gives further credence to the theory that even if active infection may have been the initial trigger, it is not always the direct cause of the ongoing symptoms.

Nevertheless, if there is strong suspicion of a coexisting active viral or bacterial carrier state, a trial course of an antibacterial, antiviral, or immune globulin is not unreasonable, and there are a few physicians who are in fact willing to undertake this. Cytomegalovirus and chlamydia are two organisms that may come into consideration since they are treatable with effective remedies. I have personally seen some persons with persistent fatigue and malaise who showed evidence of prior exposure to these organisms, and who improved significantly when empiric treatment was given targeting these organisms.

Gulf War Syndrome

Gulf War syndrome is another well-known condition where stealth infections have been considered as a potential cause. Some veterans of the first Gulf War in Iraq and Kuwait came home with illnesses and symptoms similar to those seen in CFS. In a small number of individuals specific infections were found, including a handful of cases of leishmaniasis, a rare parasitic disease. Those with the infection displayed usual signs and symptoms of this disease and responded to appropriate treatment. The vast majority of others were not proven to have infections caused by currently known germs.

The possibility was raised whether such veterans harbored unusual viruses, unusual streptococcal species, or other organisms such as microsporidia or mycoplasma. One study suggested that markers of a certain mycoplasma organism were present in the red blood cells of some of these patients. As a result, one group received extended treatment with the antibacterial antibiotic doxycycline. Some benefits were initially reported in the treated group. However, these results were not verified in other attempts to treat, and outcomes of treatment with other antimicrobials were inconsistent. Given the genetic and other variability and susceptibility of individuals, it is likely that the symptoms of Gulf War syndrome arise from several different sources and may depend on individual susceptibilities or genetic predispositions.

Once again, we should repeatedly caution against generalizing the results of these outcome studies to all persons with similar symptoms. Despite the disappointing results of the above-noted studies, some physicians may still choose to administer an empiric course of a simple antibiotic such as doxycycline, especially if there is a questionable abnormality on laboratory tests which may suggest the presence of infection.

Empiric Treatment

Most physicians believe in the judicious use of "empiric treatment." As a clinician, one can usually make a judgment about what condition is very likely, what is somewhat likely, and what is very unlikely to be the source of a person's complaints. This is not a random guess but an educated opinion based on an understanding of how particular conditions or infections behave. If an infection is strongly suspected, and if there is a simple medication that is likely to improve or eradicate the suspected infection, then the medication could be given a brief try, taking into account allergies and other potential adverse effects. The patient should be monitored for observable benefits from the treatment and the treating physician should be mindful not to overuse antimicrobials or antibiotics in view of emerging resistance of germs to antibiotics.

I have frequently encountered the need to make such a decision in cases of suspected low-grade pelvic infections of women, which are not easily proven by culture or examination. In delaying empiric treatment of such an infection, one needs to weigh the possibility of leaving the patient's infection untreated, which could be harmful to the patient and transmissible to others. Another area where empiric treatment can be cautiously considered is in cases of irritable bowel syndrome, where bacterial overgrowth of the intestines is suspected. Suspected smoldering or cycling cytomegalovirus infection could also be considered for empiric treatment.

Doxycycline Used Empirically

In the Gulf War syndrome study, the antibiotic doxycycline was chosen for empiric antibacterial treatment. This was a deliberate and well-thought-out choice based on detailed knowledge of this particular antibiotic. Though there are dozens of other anti-infective agents, it is worthwhile to highlight this particular one.

Doxycycline, originally developed in the early 1960s, is an inexpensive broad-spectrum antibacterial of the tetracycline class and is available in generic form. Teenagers often take it (or one of its close relatives, tetracycline or minocycline) for extended periods of time to treat acne.

Despite such widespread use, significant resistance of microorganisms to doxycycline has not developed. It is effective against a large number of otherwise hard-to-treat organisms (see Table 6 opposite) and also has anti-inflammatory effects. Its low cost also makes it suitable for use in impoverished areas of the world.

If the organisms or conditions in the following table are suspected to cause your ailment, a brief course of doxycycline prescribed under the supervision of your physician may be worthwhile. Some of doxycycline's benefits may be due to its anti-inflammatory properties rather than anti-infective effects, so you need to be cautious in interpreting the implications of beneficial response from treatment. Nevertheless, if some of your symptoms dramatically improve after taking the medicine, it may be a useful clue in elucidating your diagnosis.

Table 6.
Diseases and Organisms for Which
Doxycycline Is Effective Treatment*

actinomycosis	melioidosis
amebiasis	*Mycobacterium chelonei*
animal bite infections	*Mycobacterium fortuitum*
anthrax	*Mycoplasma pneumoniae*
balantidiasis	nocardiosis
brucellosis	plague
chancroid	prostatitis
Chlamydia pneumoniae	psittacosis
Chlamydia trachomatis	Q fever
cholera	relapsing fever
chronic bronchitis	Rocky Mountain spotted fever
ehrlichiosis	shigella
Enterococcus faecium	sinusitis
gonorrhea	staphylococcus, methicillin-resistant (MRSA)
granuloma inguinale	
legionella (Legionnaires' disease)	syphilis
leptospirosis	tropical sprue
Lyme disease	traveler's diarrhea
Lymphogranuloma venereum	tularemia
malaria	typhus

Doxycycline treatment also benefits rosacea, rosacea blepharitis, and early cases of rheumatoid arthritis, though specific infectious agents have not been proven to cause these conditions.

What Works?

If you were treated with an antimicrobial and subsequently you felt better, can we assume that the medicine worked? What did your improvement prove? When considering the results of medical interventions, it is useful to try to define what we mean when claiming that a medicine or therapy worked.

Many patients say that they were given a certain treatment that worked. This may include conventional treatments, alternative medicine interventions, or even homeopathic remedies. When saying this, most persons mean that whatever symptom was bothering them improved, or they felt better in general. However, we need to keep in mind that nearly four out of five medical conditions are self-limiting; in other words over time they clear up without any outside help or assistance. Was it the treatment that worked, or did the patient's condition improve due to the work of the body's defenses or the natural course of the disease or the healing process?

In scientific studies, one needs a careful definition of what is meant by the term "works." At the very least, it should mean that the remedy provided effective treatment. Does a treatment work only if it produces a certain feeling of well-being? Alternatively, does something not work if it makes you feel poorly during or right after treatment? The drug metronidazole, for example, may make you feel sick and give you a sense of nausea while you are taking it, while your bowel infection that is being treated resolves with some time-delay after you stop taking it. The same may be the case with curative radiation treatment for certain types of cancer. There are clearly "feel-good" substances that are detrimental to one's health, and there are many "bitter medicines" that help cure serious medical conditions.

We need to carefully define and refine our terms and not use antiquated descriptions. A remedy truly works if it produces a health-restoring result measurably different than in untreated or placebo-treated patients. For different conditions we need to specify the measure of the successful outcome of particular treatments above and beyond the "feel-good" criteria.

Even if successfully treated, should a person rush to tell others and encourage them to get the same treatment because it worked? Many do. Most physicians caution against such advice. Friends may have similar symptoms but may have a different condition, or a different severity of the condition, and they certainly have a different genetic makeup. Every person's treatment should be individualized. No matter how enthusiastic you are about the result of your treatment, be very cautious in convincing others to undertake the same treatment without knowing their precise diagnosis or medical condition.

Some persons try nonprescription treatments that they believe are effective in treating certain problems. When trying such remedies, patients often tell the doctor "well, at least it won't do any harm." Not quite true. Whether an ingested substance is natural or synthetic, if it truly affects the body's chemistry or physiology enough to cause some measurable effect, it is likely to have some potential adverse effect as well. Unfortunately, for nonprescription medications and health supplements, regulations do not mandate the tabulation of such adverse effects, even though they are known to exist.

One should also avoid the notion that more is necessarily better, as is well known to those who have tried to take very high doses of the vitamin niacin. Even oxygen is severely harmful when given in 100 percent concentration, whereas 21 percent is necessary for life. Various interventions, including herbs, high colonics, acupuncture, and even chiropractic treatment, are not 100 percent hazard free.

When such remedies are expensive, patients and their practitioners will surmise that it doesn't matter if the treatment acted as a placebo, what is important is that it made the person feel better, and that alone makes it worth the cost. Ethical physicians believe that those who charge for harmless but basically worthless remedies are not acting in the patient's best interest. They do financial harm to the person in return for questionable health benefits. There are legal issues involved, too. Submitting a charge to a third party, such as an insurance company, for a treatment that is known to be ineffective is considered insurance fraud.

In scientific medicine, physicians usually believe that specific conditions should be treated with specific proven interventions. Treatment expectations need to be clearly defined. There is no universal remedy for all conditions or for maintaining health. Feel-good treatments do not necessarily enhance health. There is truth in the old adage, "The doctor treats, but nature heals" (in Latin: *Medicus curat, natura sanat*). The healing that the body produces on its own can give rise to an erroneous belief in the benefits of certain treatments that were being undertaken at the same time. Cynics sometimes say: fortunately many medical problems improve despite the treatment administered!

Is there a role for self-help? Yes. Although treatment of complex medical conditions is best done with the help of experts, you should certainly take responsibility for your own health. This is not the same as treating yourself. There is difference between treatment of diseases and managing one's own health, just as there is a difference between handling day-to-day finances and making complicated investment decisions. In many simple cases self-diagnosis and treatment work. Most persons have a fair instinct for knowing when they should see a doctor and when they don't have to.

In complex cases, directing your own health care is generally inadvisable. When flying, some might feel safest flying their own aircraft. However, when navigating uncharted airspace, with rare exception, most of us would recommend relying on an experienced pilot and collaborating with the pilot to reach your destination. Remember the saying, "A physician who treats himself has a fool for a patient." In other words, even doctors believe that they must find a trusted, objective diagnostician to help solve their complicated or perplexing medical condition.

Need for Further Studies

There are no simple rules or simple answers. In treating stealth germs both short term and long term, there are many uncertainties and questions. There is a need for many more well-designed scientific outcome studies to help us make objective decisions. Some studies are currently being performed, but some may never be undertaken. For now, physicians have to individualize decisions, while using their best judgment and best educated guesses. In this way we can make prudent decisions about treatment in order to produce the best results for the physical, mental, and financial benefit of our patients.

Before going on to the general principles of protecting ourselves against infections and contagious diseases, let us revisit the emerging role of probiotics in protecting us from certain infectious conditions or against complications that may arise from their treatment.

The Use of Probiotics in Treatment and Prevention

New information is emerging about a particular approach to the management of certain complications of infections, and about protecting oneself against other infections. This area of interest is the use of prebiotics and probiotics.

Prebiotics are defined as foods containing nondigestible ingredients that when consumed provide a beneficial physiological effect by selectively stimulating the favorable growth or activity of some of the native resident bowel bacteria, primarily bifidobacteria. For that reason such foodstuffs are sometimes called "bifidogenic factors." They contain substances known as oligosaccharides and inulins.

Of course, even natural foods are not free of side effects, as we all know from eating prunes or beans. When ingesting such foods, more is not always or necessarily better. Overuse of prebiotic foods may produce bloating and other symptoms that can mask medical conditions or hamper their resolution during treatment. However, the judicious use of prebiotic nutrients under certain circumstances may help protect the microbial balance within the gastrointestinal system and the rest of the body.

Probiotics are live microorganisms that confer a health benefit when administered in adequate amounts. They are generally ingested to aid the restoration of the normal bacterial flora of the intestine, and may also provide some benefit in protecting the flora in other areas of the body. When there is suspicion that medical problems or medicines have disrupted the normal flora of a patient's gut, the use of probiotics is advised by many physicians. The use of probiotics in other conditions is being investigated. Probiotic preparations are available without a prescription.

Which Organisms Are Probiotics?

Microbes used as probiotics are not members of the normal flora of the body. They are a group of nonpathogenic live microorganisms of low virulence. Bacteria of the *Lactobacillus* and *Bifidobacterium* species are the most noteworthy. These are the some of the microbes that convert milk into cheese and yogurt by fermentation. They use sugar as their food source and produce lactic acid. However, not all lactobacillus bacteria found in all yogurts are equally beneficial.

Eating yogurt is widely believed to be of some health benefit to persons in general, and especially those taking antibiotics. Is it some particular organisms in yogurt that are healthful, or is it some other ingredient in yogurt that is beneficial? Should everyone eat a serving of yogurt every day, or should they do so only when sick or taking certain medicines? Most yogurts contain *Lactobacillus acidophilus*, an organism of uncertain benefit. However, some yogurts contain *Lactobacillus reuteri*, *Lactobacillus bulgaricus*, or *Lactobacillus rhamnosus* GG, which seem to have more demonstrable benefits.

Lactobacillus GG, when administered in capsules, may help prevent or shorten the duration of certain diarrheal illnesses, especially childhood diarrhea caused by rotavirus infection. It may also shorten the course of diarrhea experienced by persons taking antibacterial antibiotics, and also appears to have a role in preventing and treating food allergies and childhood eczema. *Bifidobacterium infantis* helps improve the symptoms of irritable bowel syndrome.

Some other organisms that are considered to have potential benefit as probiotics are *Streptococcus thermophilus*, *Enterococcus faecium*, and a harmless form of E. coli. The yeast *Saccharomyces boulardii* also has potential as a probiotic.

How Do Probiotics Work?

Probiotic organisms, when ingested in capsules, remain alive as they slip past the acid of the stomach and digestive juices of the upper intestines. They find their way to the large bowel, interestingly without stopping to colonize the normally germ-free small intestine (likely due to the inhospitable environment). Even in the colon they do not take up permanent residence, since they are not normal inhabitants of the gut. Instead, they temporarily compete with the bacteria that are already there, and with other bacteria that also don't belong. After the probiotic treatment stops, the normal bacteria of the colon return to their previous levels. The precise details of how this works are not entirely known. Nevertheless, a partial understanding of their beneficial effect is emerging.

Evidently, probiotics help out the normal flora when it has been damaged by disease or medicines. They do this partly by acting as substitutes for the healthy flora. They appear to work by outcompeting pathogenic organisms for the nutrients the pathogens would normally use to grow. By producing various acids, they increase the acidity in the intestines, which inhibits the growth of pathogenic bacteria. There is also evidence that they modify the toxins produced by pathogens, or modify toxin receptors found in the gut wall. They may also help stimulate immune responses to pathogens.

For those curious about scientific detail: The organism *Bifidobacterium* has been shown to destroy the receptor site for the toxins produced by the diarrhea-causing organism *Clostridium difficile*. The yeast *Saccharomyces boulardii* rapidly colonizes the bowel without altering the normal bacterial gut flora. It is then cleared from the colon when ingestion is discontinued. It blocks the receptor site for *Clostridium difficile* toxin. *Lactobacillus* GG increases the numbers of cells that secrete immunoglobulin A and other immune globulins in the intestinal mucosa. It also stimulates the local release of a protective compound called interferon, which is normally produced by the immune system. This microbe itself also produces an antimicrobial substance that inhibits the growth of several bacteria. As such, ingestion of such probiotics at certain times actually modifies both immune-enhancing and immune-suppressing mechanisms in the gut. Probiotics in the intestinal tract may physically or chemically prevent adhesion of pathogenic bacteria to the bowel wall.

Prevention in General

Regardless of the mechanism by which probiotics work, some outcome studies are indicating that these microorganisms are useful in helping the body overcome infections of mucosal surfaces such as the gut, vagina, and possibly the respiratory tract. They are most useful in protecting the gut, but also offer protection against vaginal bacterial and yeast problems. In children, formulas containing probiotics have been shown to reduce the incidence of diarrhea caused by viruses. Specifically, *Lactobacillus* GG has been shown to shorten the duration of diarrhea caused by rotavirus in children. In adults, probiotics are beneficial when given during gastrointestinal infections caused by *Clostridium difficile*, a pathogen that sometimes overruns the gut during antibacterial treatment given for other infections.

One study found that the probiotic *Escherichia coli* Nissle 1917 reduced the number of relapses of ulcerative colitis (a noninfectious, inflammatory bowel disease) and improved persistent inflammatory complications in a small pouch of the intestine left behind after surgery for ulcerative colitis. A study of a group of women with irritable bowel symptoms reportedly demonstrated a lessening of abdominal pain and discomfort over a four-week course of treatment with *Bifidobacterium infantis* (sold under the brand name Align).

The benefit of probiotics in modifying a condition called non-alcoholic fatty liver disease (the deposition of fat in the liver caused by conditions other than alcohol use) is also being investigated. The initial benefit observed from such treatment is explained by the interesting idea that the overgrowth of certain bacteria that naturally produce ethanol by fermentation may play a role in perpetuating fatty liver in certain individuals.

An interesting trial of a completely different class of probiotic agents is the investigational use of the eggs of the pig whipworm (*Trichuris suis*) in treating inflammatory bowel disease. Use of a preparation of these eggs has been reported to reduce disease activity in patients with active inflammation of the bowel caused by ulcerative colitis and Crohn's disease. However, such benefits remain to be confirmed. Proof is far from conclusive for the use of probiotics in various other conditions and circumstances, but results are accumulating and interesting, as tabulated in the August 2007 edition of *The Medical Letter*.

Cautions

As is true with all medical interventions, probiotics should not be used indiscriminately. Results of focused studies should not be generalized to all persons and all conditions. While there is small possibility of side effects, there have been no thorough studies of persons taking probiotics regularly over extended periods. Also, not all brands or preparations of probiotics contain the same organisms, or are prepared and packaged with the same care regarding possible contaminants. There may be differences in the survival or the organisms in the capsules on the shelf or as they travel through the gut, or the dispersal of the organisms when released from the capsules.

Even more important, the safety of using these live agents in those with severe immune deficiencies or those on chemotherapy will need to be specifically addressed. There are reports of serious infections caused by the live probiotic organisms in highly immunosuppressed and critically ill patients. As I have cautioned several times, the treatment of such individuals is outside the scope of this book. Their management has many special considerations.

Which Probiotics to Take and When?

When using probiotics, just as when using any medicinal substances, one should seek advice from someone knowledgeable in the field—preferably not exclusively from salespersons. Since this mode of treatment is not regulated by the Food and Drug Administration or other regulatory agencies, you should be especially cautious about advertised claims. Even though there is small likelihood of medical harm, there could still be some unforeseen problems caused by the indiscriminate and excessive use of these organisms. As with all medical interventions, benefits in one circumstance cannot and should not be generalized to all persons, healthy or ill, with all conditions. Information about probiotics may be verified through various sources, including responsible agencies such as the International Scientific Association for Probiotics and Prebiotics (www.isapp.net).

If one is actively taking antibiotics, the ingestion of the probiotics should be separated by a couple of hours from the time antibiotics are being taken, since antibiotics (or antifungals in the case of *Saccharomyces*) will "treat" most of these organisms and often render them ineffective.

Suggestions

Who should take probiotics and when? If you are healthy, should you take probiotics regularly as prevention? Probably not, but there is no standard recommendation at this time. However, many physicians believe that it is reasonable and useful to take probiotics when you are receiving antibiotics or as you finish taking antibiotics for treatment of an infection or if you have some of the other conditions, such as the bowel problems described above.

In those with chronic gastrointestinal complaints who have otherwise normal immunity and where other treatable conditions have been addressed, an empiric trial of probiotics may prove to be useful. It has not yet been determined how long the treatment should continue, but it likely should be taken for a limited period of time, such as a few weeks. Whether one should take probiotics all the time if one has ongoing gastrointestinal abnormalities remains to be determined. Be alert to new information in this field. The use of probiotics is a developing and evolving story.

Are there other more general measures available for protecting ourselves in our war with the microbial world? Let us explore that in the next chapter.

8. Prevention

How to Protect Ourselves: A Brief History of the War on Infectious Diseases

As we examine various measures in the prevention and treatment of stealth infections, it is interesting to look back at some recent history as it relates to the management and treatment of infections in general. In fact, our ability to truly treat infectious diseases is only about seventy-five years old.

Few of us remember that less than one hundred years ago, at the time of the great influenza epidemic of 1918, there were no antibacterials, no antivirals, no antifungals, and only a few vaccines. At that time, even in developed countries, infectious diseases caused "natural selection" among the population. Anyone with a marginal immune system, or a condition such as diabetes that weakened the immune response, succumbed to deadly infections.

The average life expectancy in the United States was approximately 47 in 1900. This was due in part to high mortality from infectious childhood diseases and other infections in adults, such as typhus, diphtheria, pneumonia, tuberculosis, and urinary infections. The influenza pandemic of 1918 caused well over 20 million deaths worldwide (some estimates give the toll at around 50 million). In 1926 the popular movie star Rudolph Valentino died at age 29 from a simple case of pneumonia. Tuberculosis (TB), then known as consumption, was a leading cause of death. TB sanitariums were present in many communities to warehouse and isolate the ill. Syphilis was also an untreatable sexually transmitted disease that could remain in your system forever and mark you for life.

By the time of the Great Depression and the advent of Social Security in the United States in the mid-1930s, life expectancy had improved to about 60 years as the result of public health measures and the development of a few vaccines to prevent the spread of infectious disease. In 1938, when my grandmother died at the age of 38 from a simple kidney infection, there were still no antibiotics to save her or anyone else's life (today she would have been "cured" within the first day of a few-day course of a simple antibiotic).

The treatment of infectious diseases took a giant leap forward with the invention of sulfa antibiotics, and soon afterward the arrival of penicillin (which was rediscovered after being originally identified in the research laboratory in 1928). During World War II, American soldiers no longer died of simple wound infections—they carried antibiotics that were effective treatment against many bacterial infections. Soon there were more antibiotics, and most bacterial infections became treatable, along with the dreaded and frequently deadly tuberculosis. Within a generation, as a result of these advances, the average life expectancy in the United States rose an additional twenty years. This remarkable thirty-year rise in average life expectancy to over 77 within less than a century, largely due to the control of infectious diseases, is a health advance unlikely to be repeated in the future.

New vaccines were being developed at a rapid pace, including the polio vaccine, along with vaccines against measles, mumps, rubella, meningitis, and more recently against hepatitis A, hepatitis B, human papillomavirus, and *Varicella zoster*. Smallpox was being eradicated from the world (fully accomplished by 1980) through public health measures and vaccination. The accelerating speed of all these advances led to the enthusiastic declaration by the Surgeon General of the United States in 1967 that the "war against infectious diseases has been won."

This announcement was not lost on the public. It generated enthusiasm, but also a certain complacency about infections. We let our guard down. There was reduced concern about sexually transmitted diseases, including the dreaded syphilis and gonorrhea, because these infections were considered fixable with a single shot of medicine or a short course of antibiotics. If you were a teenager with acne, no problem! Staying on antibiotics for months or even years would bring it under control and keep your skin looking pretty. Pneumonia and tuberculosis became easily treatable conditions. Infections, whether sexually transmitted or not, were considered to be an inconvenient nuisance to be quickly corrected and fixed, with little need for further consideration.

However, the announced victory rapidly began to crumble. To paraphrase Mark Twain, the report of the death of infectious diseases was greatly exaggerated. The emergence of AIDS threw ice water on unprotected sex. Suddenly persons with cold sores discovered that they carried a virus, which could not be eradicated from the body even with the best antimicrobials. Herpes could be sexually transmitted to an intimate partner by "shedding," even by persons without active symptoms. Intravenous drug users were found with hepatitis C in their blood, a previously unknown strain of the virus. Tuberculosis reemerged worldwide after becoming resistant to previously effective antibiotic treatment. New deadly infections such as Legionnaires' disease, SARS, Ebola virus, and avian influenza continue be serious threats to otherwise healthy persons. There is no effective treatment for several of these dangerous infections.

Four decades after the surgeon general's enthusiastic 1967 report, we know better than to think that the fight against infectious diseases is over. Anthony Fauci, of the National Institute of Allergy and Infectious Diseases, said it best: "It is now clearer than ever that the human species is in the midst of a war with microbial world, a resilient foe that will never be completely defeated." Many of the especially dangerous organisms are viruses, for which there are few effective treatments. We cannot let our guard down. We need to take a good look at how we can protect ourselves not only against stealth infections, but against infections in general.

Preventive Action Against Stealth and Other Infections

Control and prevention of stealth infections can add immeasurably not only to the length but, more important, to the quality of our lives. What do we need to do to protect ourselves and others against stealth germs and other infections?

There are both general and specific measures. The spread of infections depends on the relationships between the microorganisms, their hosts, and the environment. The risk of exposure for each of us depends on our own environment: our location, travels, dietary and other habits, sexual activity, individual susceptibilities, and so on. Furthermore, preventive action needs to be specifically tailored once we know what particular germs we are dealing with. Let us examine some general helpful principles that apply to protection against infections in general.

The Body on Autopilot

Fortunately we don't need to constantly and consciously direct or support our body's day-to-day response against every germ that lands on our body's surfaces. A remarkable feature of the human body is how well it is designed to survive! This is true for most of its functions, and is especially true in protecting itself against infections.

Our body's defenses are designed to be on "autopilot," and generally the body does an excellent job of protecting itself at all times if we give it a chance. (This consideration pertains to those with a basically normal immune system. Those born with severe immune deficiencies or those who acquire immune deficiencies require ongoing active interventions, and their management is beyond the scope of this book.) Despite widespread belief in the power of various nutritional supplements to significantly enhance the general workings of the immune system, the truth is that it is difficult to measurably improve the natural day-to-day workings of a healthy immune system by artificial means. Even highly effective vaccines enhance only small, specific parts of our immunity and not our immunity in general.

Doctors often hear their patients say "my immunity is down" or that that certain substances they took "improved my immunity." The doctor must question: What assessment has been made to come to that conclusion? The immune system is extremely complex, having humoral, cellular, and other components, and there is no known single ingestible remedy that enhances the workings of the entire system.

However, even if one's immune system is normal, and has received the usual recommended vaccinations, one cannot depend on the autopilot to do all the work without some prudent behavior on part of the "pilot." The pilot of an aircraft should not deliberately fly into severe turbulence or into the eye of a hurricane, no matter how sturdy the plane is, or even if it has an excellent autopilot. We cannot foolishly expose ourselves to overwhelming numbers of infectious invaders, even if we have a good or even superior natural immune system. We should exercise common sense and well-known precautions.

Simple Suggestions from Kindergarten

The title of a popular book states, *All I Really Need to Know I Learned in Kindergarten.* The same could be said of the knowledge needed to protect against infections. Most us remember the simple rules from our childhood: "Wash your hands," "Brush your teeth," "Keep your nose clean," "Use common sense," "Stay alert and you won't get hurt," and "Cleanliness is next to godliness." While this last statement may be concerned with morality, it also has basic health implications. The traditions of the ancients who extolled the virtues of cleanliness (purity) in life are reinforced by medical findings such as those of hand-washing pioneer Dr. Semmelweis, understanding about diseases spread by substandard hygiene, and modern evidence about sexually transmitted diseases.

The Practice of Good Hygiene

Everyone agrees that we need good basic hygiene. The word "hygiene" is used in many contexts, but generally refers to activites, actions, and practices that promote and protect health and cleanliness. The word "sanitary" is another term that is used to describe practices relating to health, and is also used to indicate being free from filth or pathogens that endanger health. The definition of these terms is not as clear as one would hope. Nevertheless, it is evident that we are well advised to exercise sanitary and hygienic practices and considerations in our personal as well as public life.

The opposite is certainly also true: Practice poor hygiene, expose yourself to infectious substances and persons, be promiscuous without protection, and you place yourself and your family at risk for developing acute and chronic medical problems.

Current evidence supports most traditional beliefs in the value of cleanliness and hygiene. Washing our body's surfaces with ordinary soap and water, especially after everyday exposure to various germs, is still an excellent general practice. Periodic hand washing is a proven measure in reducing the spread of common infections such as colds and skin bacteria. Hand washing by professional medical staff in the health-care setting has been repeatedly shown to be a critically important measure in reducing the spread of germs in the hospital or medical office. Unexpected factors, such as artificial fingernails, have been found to counteract these benefits by increasing the likelihood of harboring and transmitting infections in hospitals.

Health-care agencies promote prudent principles of hand hygiene. Hands should be washed when dirty and before eating. Hands should be washed after visiting the bathroom, especially after a bowel movement. One should not cough or sneeze into the hands. Persons should not put their unwashed fingers into their eyes, nose, or mouth. Physicians and health-care professionals should scrub their hands for at least fifteen seconds with soap or with an alcohol-based rub. Surprisingly, antibacterial soaps offer no special added benefit, and trying to fully sterilize your home or office is generally fruitless. Clean, yes; sterile, no.

Prevent Exposure

Remarkably, the body does very well to protect itself against the ordinary levels of germs that are normally around us. However, in protecting ourselves against true contagion, we have to avoid exposure to excessive numbers of pathogenic organisms. What number is excessive? It depends in part on the virulence of the germs. Even for particular germs there is no ironclad number or rule, as we noted in chapter 2.

In general we should avoid drinking significant amounts of contaminated water, eating contaminated foods, and avoid direct inoculation of certain germs into our unprotected tissues, such as by using dirty needles. We should cook our food thoroughly and filter or otherwise purify water of questionable purity. Such routine vigilance most often gives sufficient protection against germs that are only moderately virulent.

We need to be much more cautious in avoiding exposure to "killer" germs of exceptional virulence such as cholera or Ebola virus. In case of an outbreak of such an infection, we need to avoid areas where there are persons with the disease. If we need to be present, we should use protective clothing or other gear. Health-care workers in hospitals generally wear protective gloves, masks, and garbs when caring for patients with tuberculosis, influenza, or antibiotic-resistant or highly virulent infectious organisms.

Equally important to protecting ourselves from infectious organisms is the protection of others. What should we do to keep from passing infections on? Washing with soap and water and sexual hygiene are cornerstones. When you are sick, other measures are obvious: Cover your mouth—but preferably not with your hands—when coughing or sneezing. Those with open sores on their lips, mouth, genitals, or elsewhere should avoid touching others, especially after having touched or scratched their own skin sores.

Prevention is complicated by the fact that many persons are asymptomatic carriers of germs, especially those in the stealth germ category. This is one significant danger of stealth germs! Asymptomatic carriers may have colonies of contagious germs in their mouth or near their genitalia or pelvis. These germs are present in small numbers so that they don't cause any noticeable or visible symptoms, yet may be shed and transmitted to others. Even if an eruption forms, such as in the case of herpes simplex, the shedding of the microorganism may have already started a few days before the eruption and may continue for weeks after the symptomatic eruption clears. In other cases shedding of the infectious organism from body surfaces, or presence of the organisms in body fluids or secretions, may continue throughout the year.

This is why sexual hygiene such as using condoms, and using prudent measures to avoid exposure to contaminated body fluids or skin is paramount not just in certain cases, but in every case where transmission of infection is even remotely possible. At all times and under all circumstances it is our obligation to protect ourselves and our future health, as well as the health of our partners, friends, and casual contacts.

More specific preventive measures depend on one's particular environment. In this regard, we need to know the enemy, and know which germs are in our environment or neighborhood. We also need to know what germs we may encounter on foreign travel. Public health agencies have health advisories for those traveling to or residing in certain areas of the world. Some advisories apply to urban areas of industrialized countries, yet others apply in rural areas, malaria-infested areas, areas where sanitation has broken down, or for individuals traveling during certain seasons. The U.S. Centers for Disease Control and Prevention (CDC) makes available specific advisories for protection against various endemic infections that are present at a given time in various areas of the world. You can find up-to-date information on their Web site at www.cdc.gov. Travel vaccinations or prophylactic antibiotics are cornerstones of such protection.

Vaccinations

The CDC generally recommends updating certain vaccinations for adults traveling to areas of the world where there might be endemic diseases. Most of us have received the standard vaccinations during childhood. However, as adults, many of us forget to update them, unless we are in the military or in the health professions. Fortunately, in most cases our body continues to maintain immunity against the large variety of common or uncommon germs we encounter daily. If we encounter only small numbers of the germs, the body's immunity will generally have adequate defenses. We do need periodic booster shots for some of the vaccines, such as tetanus and diphtheria.

There are clearly germs such as influenza, whose particular strains may cause a sudden overwhelming illness. Since the flu virus changes yearly, annual revaccination is recommended for those who require protection, especially the elderly. New vaccines continue to become available; most recently a vaccine was developed against the *Varicella zoster* virus, which causes shingles, and another has recently become available against human papillomavirus, which can cause cancer of the female cervix. More specific recommendations about vaccinations are outlined in the next chapter.

Other Measures

If a part of your body comes in contact with known or suspected infectious materials or tissues, wash and scrub the skin promptly with soap and water, an alcohol-containing solution, or a solution of povidone/iodine.

In addition to freshening the breath, brushing your teeth and keeping your gums healthy appear to have significant medical benefits. There is evidence that periodontal disease may contribute to various problems in distant locations within the body, including the progression of atherosclerosis and kidney disease. Mouth bacteria may be the source of infection of heart valves (in the form of bacterial endocarditis) in persons with even minor heart valve abnormalities. During teeth cleaning and certain other dental procedures, bacteria from the gums may be pushed into the bloodstream. As a result, persons with heart valve problems are advised to take antibiotics right before these dental procedures. Circulating bacteria can also lodge on artificial substances within the body, such as artificial joints. Therefore, antibiotics are usually given to such patients prior to dental procedures or other procedures that may cause bacteria to circulate in the blood.

Keep your nose clean, and don't pick your nose! We learned this from parents or grandparents for a good reason. The nasal passage of many persons becomes colonized and overrun by the skin bacteria *Staphylococcus aureus*. They can be spread from the nose to other surfaces of the body, and even to other persons. This can have very serious consequences if the Staph in question is a colony of the methycillin resistant organism, MRSA. If bacteria from the nose enter the bloodstream through a sore in the nose, then infection may spread to distant parts of the body. Keeping your nose free of staphylococcus may reduce the chance of developing the serious infection called osteomyelitis, which is caused by "seeding" of the bones via the blood by germs from the nasal colony. Herpesvirus can have a presence in the nose and cause periodic sores. If you have sores in your nose, ask to be tested for staph and herpes. If you carry either of these organisms, avoid "rubbing noses" with others, and wash your hands routinely after touching your nose, especially when sores are present.

When engaging in contact more intimate than rubbing noses, we should practice meticulous sexual hygiene. Many infections can be sexually transmitted. Most of us are aware of the possibility of acquiring AIDS, herpes, syphilis, and gonorrhea via sexual contact, but chlamydia, trichomonas, hepatitis, and even mononucleosis can be transmitted by intimacy. Mechanical barriers such as condoms reduce the chances but are not foolproof in preventing the transmission of such infections.

Transferring normal bodily flora from one part of the body to another can sometimes create problems even in absence of outside organisms. "Honeymoon cystitis" is often the first bladder infection a young woman ever develops, and is common enough to be noted by this name even in medical circles. One needs to be prudent in limiting the transmission of various germs from mouth to genitalia and vice versa, or from bowel to genitalia and vice versa. There are certain hazards to introducing bowel bacteria into the pelvis, or mouth bacteria onto the urogenital tract, or certain pelvic bacteria into the mouth. During pregnancy even more care should be taken to avoid transmitting infections to the female pelvic area.

In considering further protective measures, we should remember not to jump to simple conclusions based solely on logical principles. Medicine and health are "logical" if you know all the rules, but the rules are so complex as to be overwhelming, hence we need to turn to proven information rather than just logic.

Check Your Immunity

What if it appears to you that you are getting too many infections? How many is too many? In other words, what is normal?

Minor infections are common. Children, especially those in school, may develop half a dozen to a dozen minor colds or infections per year.

Adults in close proximity to young children will often catch about half of these infections. This pattern is considered normal in young families.

Naturally, persons with certain serious underlying medical problems have increased susceptibility to infections. This is the case in those with diabetes and also applies to persons who have had their spleen removed. These persons are usually advised to receive certain extra vaccinations (such as Haemophilus, meningococcus, pneumococcus) in addition to those routinely given to others without this problem.

If you do not have the above medical problems and are generally healthy, but seem to be getting unusual, frequent, or severe infections, consider asking for a blood test to check the levels of immune globulins in your blood. If you have a true deficiency of these immune globulins, administration of remedies such as injections of gamma globulin are available.

The chemical part of the immune system is only a small part of our defenses. Previously mentioned deficiency of secretory IgA in our surface-fluids is a common finding. Doctors generally don't test for this, since there is no remedy. Nevertheless, there are tests to check for this particular deficiency in the saliva or body fluids (commercially produced kits are available). Deficiencies of our cellular immunity would need to be documented by other tests, primarily skin tests and certain blood cell counts. Those with unusual, severe, and frequent infections should consider a test for human immunodeficiency virus (HIV), or have other tests to check the response of their chemical and cellular immunity.

Adequacy of Treatment

If you are found to have an infection, it is important to treat the infection properly. Sometimes insufficient dosage of an antimicrobial medication, or inadequate length of treatment, results in repeated or recurring infections. You may not be acquiring a new infection each time; you may be having relapses of the original one.

A simple yeast infection can be treated with a single dose of medication. One day of treatment is also available for the ulcer bacteria. A single dose of antibiotic is used to protect susceptible individuals against bacteria that get into the blood during dental work. Bladder infection in women can usually be treated with three to five days of antibiotics. However, other infections, such as true kidney infections, or prostate infections in men, require longer treatment to prevent recurrence. Sinus infections may need several weeks of treatment to be thoroughly eradicated. If you were exposed to tuberculosis you will need up to several months of treatment with antibiotics before the germs are reliably eradicated from your system.

Length-of-treatment decisions are not arbitrary and not determined simply by how quickly one feels better. The duration of recommended treatment is based on studies and observations of treated patients, where success of treatment and likelihood of eradication or recurrence have been documented. In general, when undergoing this type of treatment, you should follow evidence-based textbook recommendations suggested to you by your physician.

Other Diseases

Naturally, infections are only a small fraction of all conditions and diseases that afflict human beings, though some conditions formerly thought to be noninfectious are being attributed to germs. In this chapter we have focused primarily on protection against infections.

However, we should not neglect the rest of our health. Good general health habits are essential in preventing obesity, heart disease, circulatory problems, and high blood pressure. Certain cancers are caused by environmental exposures including personal habits such as smoking. Predisposition to certain diseases may be inherited. For now this is not something we can fix, but may be able to partly correct in the future.

Do not neglect health maintenance, even in areas not related to infections. Follow good health habits. Do not smoke tobacco. Follow the periodic screening recommendations of responsible agencies such as the American Cancer Society, the American Heart Association, and the U.S. Public Health Service to check for common and preventable medical problems and conditions.

There Is No Substitute for Common Sense

Remember, the healthy body's autopilot is a really good one. Routine maintenance is usually sufficient. Follow the usual and recommended measures for health maintenance. Going overboard is not necessary. Just as with a car, you don't need to change the oil every fifty miles or even every hundred miles. However, lubricating the chassis and changing the oil at the intervals recommended by the manufacturer is prudent in helping to protect and preserve it for the longest duration.

In health maintenance there is a fine line between healthy habits and obsession. Just where is that line to be drawn? There are no set criteria. Clearly, obsessive cleanliness beyond a certain degree confers no benefits. Sterilizing doorknobs, or one's entire home, is generally unsuccessful and is of doubtful benefit. So don't go overboard. Rely on trustworthy information, and use wisdom and common sense. If you have special conditions that necessitate heightened vigilance, then follow the recommendations of your physician or responsible health agencies.

Vaccines Against Infections and Cancer?

A little-heralded area in the prevention of infections and their serious complications is the realm of vaccinations.

In addition to the Nobel Prize for the work elucidating the role of the stealth germ *Helicobacter pylori*, another major milestone in the battle against stealth germs occurred in 2005. That year saw the announcement of the initial success of the first vaccine to protect against a cancer caused by a stealth germ. Approval by the U.S. Food and Drug Administration followed in 2006. The HPV vaccine has been shown to be effective against human papillomavirus, which causes cancer of the cervix in women.

The idea of vaccinating against cancer is a remarkable new milestone. It is estimated by the World Health Organization that up to one quarter of cancers in the developing world are triggered by a handful of (mainly) viral infections. Infections play a role in cancer of the cervix, stomach, liver, and nasal passages, as well as some lymphomas and certain forms of leukemia. These cancers develop only in a fraction of the persons who are infected and are more likely to develop in those who may have certain predisposing factors. The infectious agent is only one component of the chain of events that leads to cancer development. Nevertheless, vaccines developed against these infectious triggers may work in preventing these cancers. Based on current knowledge, it is estimated that one in ten cancers could be prevented with vaccines. Human papillomavirus vaccine is estimated to prevent three quarters of cancers of the cervix. Half of liver cancers are related to the hepatitis B virus and the existing vaccine could prevent most of these.

What Is a Vaccine?

Just what is a vaccine? And why aren't there vaccines against all infections? Could there be a vaccine against AIDS or malaria? Why does a new vaccine need to be produced for influenza every year? Why don't persons get vaccinated against smallpox anymore? (Many older persons still have the small scar on their shoulder or their thigh from smallpox vaccinations.) Why don't we all receive the same vaccinations that are given to military personnel when they go abroad? Isn't there a vaccine against tuberculosis, and if so, why isn't it used? What about reports that some day in the future there may be a vaccine against schizophrenia and cancer of the pancreas? Can several vaccinations be given on the same day, or does each one need to be given separately? Are there vaccines that contain live viruses as opposed to vaccines with "killed" viruses? Who invented vaccinations anyway?

Vaccinations stir up all these interesting questions. There are straightforward answers to most of them. I will address some of them.

Vaccines are of such fundamental importance that numerous Nobel Prizes have been awarded for work in the field. Looking back in history, the first Nobel Prize given for medicine was awarded in 1901 to Emil von Behring for the development of diphtheria antiserum. It is still given to children as part of the DPT (diphtheria-pertussis-tetanus) vaccination. The 1951 Nobel Prize in medicine went to Max Theiler for the development of a vaccine against yellow fever, and in 1954 the Nobel Prize went to John Enders, Thomas Weller, and Frederick Robbins for a culture of the poliovirus that led to the development of the successful vaccine against polio.

Other Nobel Prizes relating to infectious disease went to Robert Koch in 1905 for his study of tuberculosis (Koch's research eventually led to a tuberculosis vaccine), to Charles Laveran in 1907 for discovering the role of protozoa (such as *Giardia* or *Blastocystis*) in disease, and Charles Nicolle in 1928 for discovering the pathogenesis of typhus. In 1966 the prize was awarded to Peyton Rous and Charles Huggins for discovering that viruses cause tumors, and in 1976 to Baruch Blumberg and D. Carleton Gajdusek for their work on slow viruses, including hepatitis B, which led to a vaccine against hepatitis B.

Except for the Nobel Prize winners, those who work on vaccines are generally unheralded. They work quietly in scientific laboratories, often as a group of researchers rather than a single investigator. Only a few have been colorful enough to catch the attention of the press and the public. One such man was Jonas Salk, who competed with Albert Sabin in the development of the polio vaccine. While many of us are aware of the yearly influenza vaccinations that are available, few of us know or even think about who is involved in manufacturing the vaccine or how it is prepared—unless there is a shortfall. The HPV vaccine is certainly in the news these days, but hardly anyone knows who is responsible for its development.

Which of these many different vaccinations should a person get? Why not just get a shot against every possible infection, then be done with infections? Wouldn't it be possible to win the war on infectious diseases in this way? Great idea, but as usual, the devil's in the details.

Most physicians recommend and most persons agree to undergo a set series of vaccinations against certain diseases, especially so-called childhood vaccinations. Nevertheless, despite widespread use of vaccinations, we cannot let our guard down: these infections continue to be among us. Only one—smallpox—has been truly eradicated, and even this could resurface in an instant if someone let the virus loose from a laboratory where cultures of it are stored.

Many diseases—measles, mumps, polio, tetanus, diphtheria, and others—would return widely and become significant public health problems within a few years if we stopped vaccinating. These potential killer or crippling diseases are still a major health problem in underdeveloped parts of the world. For example, measles kills an estimated one million children worldwide annually. Even in the United States, several hundred children and an estimated 25,000 to 30,000 adults die of vaccine-preventable infections every year (mainly influenza and pneumonia). Most adults do not keep up to date with their vaccinations. Vaccinations are only for children, they think, and childhood shots are a "forgettable" unpleasant experience.

Concerns About Vaccination

Some persons are concerned that vaccines, like most medical interventions, are not free of potential side effects. However, the majority of side effects from the shots are minor and predictable: soreness, some redness, and minor bruising over the muscle or skin near the injection site. Generalized reactions such as fever, headache, or malaise are less common, and their likelihood depends on the particular vaccine.

Extremely rare, but serious and potentially fatal reactions do occur. This only happens with some, but not all, vaccines. Such reactions are extremely uncommon among the millions of children who receive vaccines annually. Are such reactions truly random chance, or do those children who develop such severe reactions have some quirk in their immune system to begin with? Perhaps they are not only reacting poorly to the vaccine, but could have reacted equally severely had they gotten the infection itself. These are important questions for which there are no definite and conclusive answers. Nonetheless, because of these rare reports, some parents refuse vaccinations for their children for fear of a possible serious complication. Unfortunately, poorly informed generalization can be the basis of prejudice, which is also true in realms outside of medicine.

Other concerns have been raised by the public about a possible link between the administration of vaccines and new-onset Type 1 diabetes in children following vaccination. Meticulous studies have proven no such association. Another concern arose about measles immunization being linked to autism. Again, no cause-and-effect relationship has been established. Nevertheless, potential adverse reactions to vaccines are being monitored, and a risk-versus-benefit determination needs to be made for each individual vaccine, old or new, and each individual recipient, young or old. Based on such considerations, some new vaccines have been withdrawn from the market.

Regardless of concerns about side effects, why is there not a vaccine for everything? Wouldn't that be the best possible weapon against infections and even cancer? To understand the answer, one needs to know how the process of vaccination works.

The History of Vaccination

The word vaccine derives from *vaccinia*, the Latin name for the infectious virus which causes cowpox. The story of the discovery of the first vaccination by Edward Jenner, an English country doctor, yields interesting insight into how vaccines work.

During an epidemic of smallpox in 1796, Jenner observed that those of his patients who worked with cattle and had previously had the mild disease of cowpox (similar to chicken pox) did not become ill with the potentially deadly smallpox, even when exposed. He surmised that if he could purposely expose persons to cowpox, the germs from the cowpox would somehow activate the body's defenses against the more dangerous smallpox germs. He tested his approach on a farmer's son, and it worked! The boy "vaccinated" with cowpox did not become ill when he was deliberately exposed to smallpox. Just as with Semmelweis, initially Jenner was the subject of skepticism and ridicule. Yet, over two centuries later, we continue to use the principles he pioneered.

One problem in developing vaccines against all infections is that, unlike cowpox and smallpox, a "harmless" animal variant does not exist of every infectious organism. Since it can be very dangerous to inoculate even small doses of live pathogens into someone who has little or no immunity to that pathogen, vaccines are usually prepared from killed pathogenic organisms or parts of such organisms. However, a closely related organism or a killed organism is often not enough to stimulate or fool the immune system into building up defenses against the true pathogen. Small doses or weakened forms of the live organism may work, but these can precipitate the actual infection in some persons, especially those with unusual susceptibilities. This is one of the reasons why vaccines are available only against a few dozen organisms and why effective vaccines against AIDS and malaria have been difficult to produce. Nevertheless, efforts continue to produce vaccines against various dangerous organisms. Synthetic processes and those derived by recombinant DNA technology are also being pursued.

Vaccines Against Noninfectious Conditions

Vaccines are beginning to be used against noninfectious processes. Pancreatic cancer cells killed by irradiation were used in a recent investigational trial to see if the body's immune system would recognize, and mount a defense against, the abnormal cancerous cells. Preliminary results indicated that this vaccine extended survival of patients following surgical removal of their pancreatic cancer.

A vaccine has been developed and tried against Alzheimer's disease, a condition characterized by the buildup of a certain abnormal protein (beta-amyloid) in the brain. The immune system of patients indeed responded by reacting against the abnormal protein. However, even though favorable results were observed in the clearance of the abnormal substance, a small percentage of patients who received the vaccine developed autoimmune encephalitis, a reaction against their own normal human brain cells, and hence this form of the vaccine was not usable.

Why Is the Vaccine Against Tuberculosis Not Used?

Even when a vaccine is available it is not necessarily used. A prime example of this is the tuberculosis vaccine. There are two reasons for this. First, the vaccine provides less than full protection. Furthermore, once the vaccine is given, the body's immune response is activated and one's tuberculosis skin test, a primary method of detecting new exposure to TB, shows positive results for the foreseeable future. In the United States, where tuberculosis is rare, vaccination is not generally given in order to preserve the value of the skin test for detecting new cases. In other areas of the world where TB is common, the vaccination is used. In those regions protection supersedes the benefit of using the skin test for detection of new cases, which can also be done in other ways.

For further information about vaccines, you should consult the Web sites of the National Center for Immunization and Respiratory Diseases (a department of the CDC) at www.cdc.gov/vaccines/ and the National Network for Immunization Information at www.immunizationinfo.org. Vaccinations will continue to evolve as an important way of protecting ourselves against serious infections and related illnesses. The role of vaccinations in the prevention of cancer may be one of the major medical accomplishments of the early 21st century! A partial list of vaccines and guidelines for vaccinations at the time of this writing are provided in the tables that follow.

Table 7. Vaccines Against Some Human Pathogens		
Infectious Agent	**Vaccine Status**	**Disease**
Bacteria		
Bacillus anthracis	available	anthrax
Bordetella pertussis	available	whooping cough
Borrelia burgdorferi	available	Lyme disease
Clostridium tetani	available	tetanus
Corynebacterium diphtheriae	available	diphtheria
Coxiella burnetii	available	Q fever
Haemophilus influenzae	available	meningitis,epiglottitis, pneumonia type b
Mycobacterium leprae	in development	leprosy
Mycobacterium tuberculosis	available	tuberculosis
Neisseria meningitidis subgroup B	in development	meningitis
Neisseria meningitidis subgroup C	available	meningitis
Salmonella typhi	available	typhoid fever
Staphylococcus aureus	in development	impetigo, toxic shock in women
Streptococcus pneumoniae	available	pneumonia, middle ear infection, meningitis
Vibrio cholerae	available	cholera
Viruses		
adenovirus	available	respiratory disease
hepatitis A	available	liver disease, cancer
hepatitis B	available	liver disease, cancer
human papillomavirus	available	cervical cancer
Influenzavirus A	available	influenza
Influenzavirus B	in development	influenza
Japanese encephalitis virus	available	brain infection
measles virus	available	respiratory infection, subacute sclerosing panencephalitis
mumps virus	available	mumps, meningitis, orchitis

poliovirus	available	polio, paralysis
rabies virus	available	rabies
rubella virus	available	German measles, fetal malformations
vaccinia virus	available	smallpox
Varicella zoster virus	available	chicken pox, shingles
yellow fever virus	available	jaundice, kidney and liver failure
Parasites		
leishmania	in development	kala-azar, tropical sores
Fungus		
Coccidioides immites	in development	lung infection
Cancer		
cervical cancer	available	against human papillomavirus
liver cancer	available	against hepatitis B

Table 8.

Pediatric and Adult Vaccines Recommended by the Advisory Committee on Immunization Practices for Routine Use in Otherwise Healthy U.S. Residents

Recommended Pediatric Immunizations

diphtheria-tetanus-pertussis (DTP) vaccine

Haemophilus influenzae type *b*

hepatitis A vaccine

hepatitis B vaccine

human papillomavirus vaccine

inactivated polio vaccine

influenza vaccine

meningococcal conjugate vaccine

measles-mumps-rubella (MMR) vaccine

pneumococcal conjugate vaccine

rotavirus vaccine

varicella vaccine

Recommended Adult Immunizations

hepatitis A vaccine (selected populations)

hepatitis B vaccine (adults at risk)

human papillomavirus vaccine (under age 26)

influenza vaccine (selected populations; over age 50 and health-care workers)

measles-mumps-rubella (MMR) vaccine

pneumococcal polysaccharide vaccine (selected populations; over age 65)

tetanus-diphtheria vaccine

varicella vaccine

Zoster (shingles) vaccine (over age 60)

**Recommended Vaccinations in the Presence
of Certain Medical Conditions**

Special suggestions are needed for vaccination in the context of conditions such as pregnancy, diabetes, heart disease, chronic pulmonary disease, chronic liver disease, congenital immunodeficiency, leukemia, lymphoma, generalized malignancy, chemotherapy with alkylating agents, antimetabolites, radiation, use of large amounts of corticosteroids, renal failure, end-stage renal disease, those on hemodialysis or receiving clotting factor concentrates, those without a spleen, including those scheduled for elective removal of the spleen, those with terminal complement component deficiencies, and those with HIV infection. Consult with your doctor about such special considerations.

Adapted from the National Center for Immunization and Respiratory Diseases, Centers for Disease Control and Prevention.

9. Conclusion

What Does the Future Hold?

Newly developed vaccines against stealth infections and cancers caused by microbes are only one of the areas in which medicine faces an exciting future. On the diagnostic front, major advances continue to enable us to detect diseases, including infections, in increasingly accurate detail. The human genome has been sequenced, and this will lead to major advances in the understanding of individual reactions and predispositions to various diseases. On the therapeutic front, pharmacological and technological advances are providing novel ways of curing and treating disease.

Even taking these advances into account, the continued threat from infectious organisms should not be underestimated. Infectious diseases continue to be a source of major problems in developing countries. The control of infectious diseases and stealth infections is going to require sustained vigilance and effort. Many attack microbes, such as influenza, are doing their best to stay a step ahead of us. There are newly emerging pathogenic organisms, constantly changing and mutating, such as bird flu and SARS.

The AIDS virus has been known for less than three decades. But where did it come from? It is believed that a virus, previously harbored by animals, evolved to leap from its animal host and was able to adapt to human beings. This is one of the mechanisms by which such new human diseases suddenly emerge. The threat of influenza and other pandemics continues to loom.

Sadly, there is also the concern of bioterrorism and how it might spread dangerous infections by deliberate action, causing the resurgence of diseases, such as smallpox, which are currently considered to be

eradicated. It is sad to realize that there are persons who seek to deliberately undo the work of a multitude of others who dedicated their lives
to the betterment of the health of their fellow human beings.

In addition to highly virulent and highly visible aggressive microbes
such as influenza, stealth germs will continue to cleverly and quietly
infect human beings, persisting in their destructive work. Even though
they don't kill their host rapidly, there is no question that over time
stealth germs can cause considerable trouble for humanity. As Dr. Siobhan
O'Connor, Associate Director of the National Center for Infectious
Diseases at the Centers for Disease Control and Prevention, stated, "It is
becoming increasingly acceptable and recognized that infections are
probably an underappreciated cause of chronic diseases." It has been my
goal to heighten awareness of some of these stealth infections as we currently understand them.

A number of catastrophic events over the last few years reminded us
how potentially fragile our defenses are when it comes to holding the
fort against infections. In refugee camps, which are necessitated by sense-
less wars or after various natural disasters, infections threaten the sur-
vivors. Even though mass epidemics did not occur, only years from now
will we fully know how many may have acquired silent stealth infections
from contaminated waters, polluted environment, and lack of basic
hygiene, even if actual exposure was only for a short time.

Unfortunately, there is an economic factor to stealth infections and
other infections as well. People of low socioeconomic means are at the
greatest risk for exposure to harmful infections. They may lack the simple tools of hygiene, access to clean food and water, or ready access to
information and resources that would help them protect themselves.
They are often hampered by poor education and even by unhelpful cus-
toms and traditions. In underdeveloped areas of the world, where educa-
tional attainment is low and public health measures and sanitation are
poor, infectious diseases are rampant. Illnesses that produce prompt and
damaging results, such as blindness due to trachoma, urinary infections
from schistosomiasis, and cases of tuberculosis, AIDS, and malaria are
widespread and highly visible. Damage from stealth diseases is less obvious

to see. The extent to which persons carry *Helicobacter pylori* in their stomachs that may develop into cancer decades later, or the extent to which the brains of individuals in polluted environments may be affected by hit-and-run stealth germs, or by germs harbored in this system for years, is much more difficult to determine.

Even in industrialized societies such as the United States, we cannot let our guard down. Intimate sexual contact can spread human papillomavirus, chlamydia, herpes, and other venereal or sexually transmitted diseases. In sexual intimacy, protection against a variety of lesser-known but equally common and troublesome infections is of paramount importance, with special regard for the protection of pregnant women and newborn infants.

An individual's susceptibility to stealth germs is compounded by genetic predisposition as well as environment. For example, rising obesity rates worldwide are leading to increasing numbers of persons with diabetes, affecting those who are genetically susceptible. Persons with diabetes are in turn more susceptible to infections. Those with blood disorders, such as sickle-cell disease, are more susceptible to some infections as well.

Of continued concern is the development of resistance by infectious organisms to antibiotics and antimicrobials. This is in part due to the remarkable adaptive power of germs and partly due to the improper use of antibiotics. As a result, a short seven decades after antibiotics were first discovered and introduced, many antibiotics are no longer effective against infectious conditions that they once easily cured. Staying one step ahead of emerging resistant organisms poses a major technological challenge.

Remarkably in our favor, human biology also spontaneously evolves. There are fascinating documented cases of rare persons who have natural immunity against AIDS, and it is possible that in areas of the world where the disease is widespread, groups of individuals may emerge who are resistant to the HIV virus. Soon there may be ways of transferring such immunity via genetic material to others.

There are many reasons for optimism. On the detection front, blood tests, PCR tests, MRI scans, CT scans, white blood cell scans, and so on, are enabling us to pin down infections lurking in hidden areas of the body. Considerable research is focused on the field of stealth infections.

On the treatment front, the first vaccine ever against a cancer is now available. New antiviral agents and other treatments are being developed against the AIDS and hepatitis viruses. There may be more antivirals and new vaccines against organisms that may be the trigger for conditions such as Type 1 diabetes or multiple sclerosis. Preventive measures or early treatment may keep such viruses from triggering the body's excessive immune reaction, often the source of much damage. Nanotechnology, genetic engineering, and stem cell research are promising new fields with exciting potential for remarkable health benefits.

In the realm of infections (as is true in general), first and foremost we need to take responsibility for our own well-being. Many simple measures continue to work remarkably well for disease prevention. Use common sense and good judgment. Wash your hands with soap and water. Cover your mouth and nose when sneezing, then go wash your hands again. Protect yourself against sexually transmitted diseases. Don't spit on the sidewalk. Be careful to protect others when you are sick. Stay at home when you are ill with an infection. Stay clear of others who have an obvious infection. Then wash your hands again.

Some infections can in fact be eliminated with such "low-tech" measures. Simple isolation of those with smallpox to prevent person-to-person contagion allowed that disease to be eradicated. This was accomplished not because there were million-dollar scanners and $1,000-per-month medications, but because knowledgeable individuals took the time and made the effort to show persons a few simple, common-sense measures. Clean drinking water is essential. Inspection of foods is beneficial. Irradiation of foods may be one way to decontaminate food supplies in areas where clean food and water are unavailable.

Information disseminated through the Internet is useful, but should be used with caution. Unedited information and promotion of questionable non-evidence-based treatments and remedies greatly dilutes and confounds the scientifically valid information available online. Technology needs to be applied with wisdom. As has been a theme of this book, both in diagnosis and treatment it is our brain that needs to get the picture. Infectious diseases change, but they also remain largely the same. Let us learn. Let us teach health information and hygiene in the public schools. Let us pass on this information from father to son and from mother to daughter. Through books such as this, let us heighten public awareness. Collaboration between public health agencies, the medical community, and educated citizens will be of paramount importance for the foreseeable future.

End of This Journey and on to the Future

It is time to conclude our journey with stealth germs. I started on a personal note, and I wish to end on a personal note. Let me close with some thoughts from one of my medical predecessors, Dr. Rexwald Brown of Santa Barbara, California, where I have had the good fortune to work for most of my career. In 1926 he wrote:

> "The highest ideal of medicine is the promotion of individual, community, and national health. . . . Collaboration between the people and the medical profession is essential to the real accomplishment of scientific medicine's greatest aim: health promotion."

I offer this book as one small step in furthering these ideals. It is also my hope to further the goal that I laid out in my first "House Calls" column in the *Santa Barbara News Press*: "In these times of information explosion, we need experts to sort out, interpret and put in perspective some of the apparently contradictory and confusing reports. I hope to be such an interpreter."

More than just being an interpreter, I hope to have passed on some useful knowledge to you, the reader. In this regard, I deviated in a small part from the Oath of Hippocrates cited in the Appendix. Part of the oath would have me declare that "I will impart a knowledge of the art (of medicine) to my own sons and to those of my teachers, and to disciples bound by a stipulation and oath, according to the law of medicine, but to none others."

In a revision of the oath for the modern world, I would like to impart my medical knowledge to all persons, rather than just a chosen few. If you, the reader, will help me, then we can work together to promote and disseminate responsible medical information useful to the public health and the health of all of our fellow human beings.

Here is to our health and to the health of future generations!

Appendix

To My Doctor

Name _____

Birthdate _____

Date _____

My chief concern is that I have _____ (symptoms)
in my _____ (body region; for example:
head, chest, abdomen, pelvis, skin).

My symptoms and how they evolved are as follows:

_____

_____

_____

_____

_____

Past medical conditions: _____

Past operations: _____

Past accidents or injuries: _____

Habits (smoking, alcohol): _____

Medicines and supplements taken: _____

Allergies: _____

Family history: _____

Miscellaneous other symptoms: _____

Questions for my Doctor

1. Could my symptoms be caused by chronic infection or colonization of my _____ by _____
   (body region)   (name of condition)
   or a condition called _____
   (name of proposed possible infectious organism)

2. If so, are there tests such as _____ to prove or disprove it, or other tests which could be done such as sedimentation rate, serum protein electrophoresis, white blood cell count, which could give clues to the presence of an infection?

3. If no proof is available, or even if my tests are negative, could I take an anti-infective _____
   (name of medicine/antibiotic/antiviral)
   "empirically" to see if my symptoms improve or go away?

4. Do you think there might be more than one process or condition—one of which is a treatable infection—in my system to explain my problems?

Doctor's Reply

It is POSSIBLE LIKELY UNLIKELY IMPOSSIBLE that you have or carry an infectious condition because _____
_____
_____

Your actual diagnosis is _____
Your treatment should be _____
If you don't get better RETURN TO SEE ME IN _____
                                            (days or weeks)
and/or SEE SPECIALIST _____

_____ , M.D.
(signed)

Glossary

AIDS

Acquired immunodeficiency syndrome is a severe disorder of the body's cell-mediated immune response. It results in increased likelihood of various opportunistic infections, and some cancers, some of which may be triggered by infections. AIDS is caused by an acquired infection with the human immunodeficiency virus (HIV).

antibacterial

A substance that destroys bacteria or interferes with and retards their growth.

antibiotic

A chemical or biologic substance that stops or inhibits the growth of various microorganisms, prevents their development, or inhibits their disease-producing action. Most often used to refer to antibacterial medicines or substances, but also sometimes to anti-fungal and anti-parasitical agents. Generally *not* used to mean anti-viral agents.

antibody

An immunoglobulin protein substance present in the blood or tissues. Antibodies are one part of the immune system which attacks, destroys, or incapacitates bacteria and neutralizes biologic poisons. Each of the numerous different immunoglobulins is produced specifically in response to a particular bacterium or toxin (antigen), and interacts only with the antigen that induced it, or with another closely related antigen.

antifungal

A substance that destroys fungi, prevents their development, or inhibits their disease-producing action.

antimicrobial

A substance that destroys microorganisms, prevents their development, or inhibits their disease-producing action.

antigen

Any biologic or biochemical substance, such as toxins, bacteria, or the cells of transfused blood and transplanted organs, that induce the production of antibodies by the immune system of the host.

antiseptic

A substance or a process that prevents or stops the spread of infectious agents.

antiviral

A substance that destroys viruses, prevents their development, or inhibits their disease-producing action.

bacterium, bacteria

Any microorganism that belongs to the biologic class named Schizomycetes. They are able to be free-living, and can colonize or produce disease in humans, animals, and plants. Bacteria vary greatly in their shape and nutritional requirements, and may be harmless, health-promoting, or pathogenic.

Blastocystis hominis

A parasitic organism of the protozoa class found in various places around the world. When ingested in the form of contaminated food or water, it can colonize the bowels and may cause loose or watery stools, gassiness, or abdominal pain. However, many persons who carry it may have essentially no symptoms, and therefore the organism has been historically considered to be non-pathogenic. If untreated, it may remain in the bowels for weeks, months, or years.

blood-brain barrier

The physiological mechanism within the capillaries of the brain that alters their permeability, so that various biochemical substances (chemicals and drugs) cannot freely enter or leave the brain tissue, while other substances are allowed to do so.

broad-spectrum antibiotic
Generally refers to an antibacterial antibiotic which has a wide range of activity against most bacteria, but not viruses, fungi, or protozoa.

carrier state
The condition whereby an individual harbors a potential disease-causing organism without showing signs and symptoms of infection, yet can be the source of infection to others.

cervix
The medical name generally used to refer to the narrow outer end ("neck") of the uterus located in the female pelvis. (Sometimes used to refer to the human neck itself.)

colonization, colony
A group of organisms which grow on a surface of the body. Such a surface may be on the outside, such as the skin, or on the inside, such as the inside surface of the stomach or the sinuses.

commensal organisms
An organism which becomes part of a symbiotic relationship, so that one species benefits from the relationship, while the other is not affected.

communicable disease
Also called contagious disease, it is transmitted between persons or species through direct contact with the individual who is infected, or indirectly through an intermediary, such as a mosquito.

computerized tomography, CT scan
Diagnostic imaging of the body's internal structures using X-rays, in which computer analysis and processing of scans made along planes through the body creates a three-dimensional image of that area of the body.

contagion, contagious
Transmission of a disease by direct or indirect contact, as in a communicable disease, or the state of carrying a disease, with the ability to transmit it to others.

culture
The growing of microorganisms or tissue cells, outside the body in an artificial environment, such as a laboratory dish or tube, which contains and provides nutrient for the growth.

dual infection
The simultaneous presence of two (or more) significant infections in the same patient.

electrocardiogram (EKG)
A recording of electrical signals from the surface of the body, which selects out and records the electric activity of the heart, used for the detection of certain (but not all) heart abnormalities.

empiric treatment
Treatment guided by experience and knowledge, rather than by direct proof provided by the results of tests.

endocarditis
Inflammation or infection of the thin membrane called the endocardium that lines the interior of the heart, including the valves of the heart.

endometriosis
A condition caused by the abnormal presence of functioning endometrial tissue outside the uterus, often in the form of cysts containing blood. It is characterized by pain and discomfort in parts of the abdomen, pelvis, or even more distant areas of the body, which cycle with menstrual periods, but do not originate from the uterus.

evidence-based medicine
Medical diagnosis and treatment based on the use of evidence of the efficacy of such diagnosis and treatment obtained by formal scientific methods and studies.

"fishing expedition"
A term used by physicians to refer to a process of diagnostic problem-solving whereby the diagnostician has no specific idea of what they are looking for. A large number of various tests is ordered to "see what will turn up."

fungus
An organism of the living species classified as Fungi. They may be single celled, or grow as branched multi-celled structures that often produce characteristic "fruiting bodies." Yeasts are one particular member of this family.

germ
A microorganism, but often used to refer particularly to a disease-causing microorganism.

humoral immunity
The component of the immune response that involves so-called plasma cells, that produce and release antibodies to a specific antigen.

immune globulins
A family of proteins in the blood, which are produced in response to specific antigens, such as bacteria or toxins. Various classes of the immune globulins include immunoglobulin A, immunoglobulin E, immunoglobulin G, and immunoglobulin M, with each class having particular roles in the immune defenses.

immune system
The integrated system of particular organs, tissues, cells, proteins, and cell products of the body that neutralize invading pathogenic organisms or substances by the process of recognizing and differentiating the body's self from other organisms, cells, and substances that "do not belong."

immunocompetent
Possessing the ability of the body to mount a normal immune response when exposed to an antigen.

immunocompromised

Lacking the ability to mount a normal immune response, usually because of disease, malnutrition, or treatments that suppress the functioning of the immune system.

infection

The process of having germs overrun or invade a region of the body, and in the process produce inflammation or injury to these bodily tissues, which progresses to damage or disease through a variety of biological mechanisms.

infectious disease

A harmful medical or biological condition caused by a pathogenic microorganism.

infest

In the way of a parsite, to inhabit or overrun an area of the body in numbers large enough to be irritating, or truly harmful.

inflammation

A localized protective reaction of tissue triggered by injury, chemical or biologic irritants or infection, most often characterized by pain, redness, and swelling. Low-grade inflammation may not produce observable outward signs, and is identified by characteristic microscopic features of the inflamed tissue.

interstitial cystitis

A persistent inflammatory condition of currently undetermined cause, that affects the lining and the muscular tissue of the bladder.

invasive

Refers to the tendency for an infection or a tumor to spread into another tissue, especially into healthy tissue. In another context, the term *invasive procedure* refers to a medical procedure in which a part of the body is penetrated, such as by incision or puncture.

irritable bowel syndrome
Persistent motility disorder of the intestines, often characterized by spasmodic pains, diarrhea, or constipation. Can be due to various causes; and low-grade infections as a potential cause or contributing factor may be overlooked.

lymphocytes
Cells of the white blood cell category, formed by tissues in the lymph nodes, spleen, thymus, and tonsils. They are a key component of the immune system in the form of two specific cell types, B cells and T cells.

magnetic resonance imaging (MRI)
Imaging technique for obtaining highly detailed images of internal structures of the body without the use of radiation and X-rays. The images are created by computer processing, using information from radio-frequency signals modified by magnetic fields aimed at and recorded from the body.

normal flora
The microorganisms that inhabit a bodily organ or part of normal healthy individuals.

opportunistic infection
Microorganisms that rarely if ever cause disease in persons with a normal immune system, yet cause serious disease in patients whose immunity is compromised by various illnesses or treatments.

outcome study
Study of the results of treatment in a group of patients treated with a certain medication or intervention, with the aim of documenting both short- and long-term benefits or detrimental effects of the treatment. Serves as the foundation of evidence-based medicine.

ova and parasites test
Laboratory test that examines fecal material or other bodily fluid to look for evidence of worms or other parasites that may be present in the body. The test searches for their eggs (ova), or for the parasites themselves or their fragments.

pathogen
A disease-causing microorganism such as a bacterium, virus, or fungus, but is sometimes used to refer to any other disease-causing substance.

perineum
Term used to refer to the portion of the pelvis occupied by urogenital passages and the rectum, whose boundaries are the pubic arch in the front, the tailbone in the back, and part of the hipbone along the sides. It is also often used to refer to the surface region between the scrotum and the anus in males, and between the back end of the vulva and the anus in females.

prebiotic
Foods, which have ingredients that do not digest fully, but pass through the intestines to the colon, where they produce a beneficial effect by providing residual nutrient substances, which promote the growth of some of the local resident "beneficent" bowel bacteria, such as bifidobacteria.

prednisone, prednisolone
Synthetic steroid compounds similar to cortisone or hydrocortisone that are used as strong anti-inflammatory or immunosuppressive agents in the treatment of various conditions.

prion
Proteinaceous infectious particle whose mode of action is only partly understood. It is composed entirely of proteins, and is believed to be a cause of several contagious conditions.

probiosis
An association of two organisms that promotes and improves the life processes of both.

probiotic
Live microorganisms that provide a health benefit to the host or the recipient.

prostate-specific antigen (PSA) blood test

A blood test that measures a particular chemical produced by the male prostate gland. Elevated levels may indicate the presence of inflammation of the prostate, enlargement of the prostate, or cancer of the prostate. The antigen is specific for the prostate, but not specific for particular conditions such as cancer of the prostate.

protozoa

Any of a group of single-celled organisms, differentiated from bacteria. Giardia, malaria, and amoebas are notable members of the protozoa family.

pus

A name for a congregation of white blood cells, often used to refer to visible amounts.

receptor

A site or molecular structure on the surface or interior of a cell that allows the binding of biochemical substances such as drugs, hormones, antigens, or neurotransmitters.

serum

The fluid portion of the blood which remains after blood cells are removed.

stealth germ

An infectious microorganism that enters the body and may stay in one's body for extended periods of time and cause minimal or no symptoms, or symptoms generally not interpreted as signs or indications of an infection, yet be the cause of various conditions and serious diseases previously or otherwise attributed to noninfectious causes.

strain

A particular subtype of a pathogenic microorganism that may be more or less virulent than other subtypes of the same organism.

superficial

In medical context, this refers to being on or near the surface of the body.

symbiosis, symbiotic
An association of mutual benefit between two or more different organisms of different species, though it may not benefit each member equally.

symptom
A feeling or observation experienced by a person as a change from normal sensation, function, or appearance, which often, but not necessarily indicates disease or a significant disorder.

vaccine
A preparation of a weakened, altered, or killed pathogenic microorganism, which upon administration to a host stimulates the production of antibodies by the host against the pathogen to provide eventual immunity against the pathogen, but does not produce severe infection in the process.

virulence
How powerful a particular disease-causing germ is in its ability to cause disease. In animal models, attempts to quantitate virulence are done by measuring how many of the organisms it takes to cause disease in 50 percent of the hosts, or how many organisms are required to kill at least 50 percent of the hosts.

virus
Submicroscopic parasites which invade the cells of humans, plants, animals, and bacteria, and often but not always cause disease. They are not considered true living organisms, since they consist primarily of a core of RNA or DNA surrounded by a protein cover, and are incapable of replicating without a host cell.

white blood cell
Also called white corpuscles or leukocytes, these are the colorless or white cells in the blood that have a nucleus and cytoplasm and help protect the body from infection and disease. There are various subtypes, including lymphocytes, monocytes, neutrophils, eosinophils, each with a different role in the workings of the immune system.

yeast

A single-celled fungus of the *Saccharomyces* category, which reproduces by budding. Yeasts are commonly known for their capability to ferment carbohydrates.

Zenker's diverticulum

Also called a *hypopharyngeal diverticulum*. A pouch or sac that forms just below the vocal cords from the inner lining of the esophagus. It may trap festering foodstuffs.

Oath of Hippocrates

I swear by Apollo the physician, Æsculapius, and Hygieia, and Panacea, and all the gods and goddesses, that, according to my ability and judgment, I will keep this Oath and this stipulation:

To reckon him who taught me this Art equally dear to me as my parents, to share my substance with him and to relieve his necessities if required; to regard his offspring as on the same footing with my own brothers and to teach them this Art, if they shall wish to learn it, without fee or stipulation. By precept, lecture and every other mode of instruction, I will impart a knowledge of the Art to my own sons and to those of my teachers, and to disciples bound by a stipulation and oath according to the law of medicine, but to none others.

I will follow that system of treatment which, according to my ability and judgment, I consider for the benefit of my patients, and abstain from whatever is deleterious and mischievous. I will give no deadly medicine to anyone if asked, nor suggest any such counsel; furthermore, I will not give to a woman an instrument to produce abortion.

With purity and holiness I will pass my life and practice my Art. I will not cut a person who is suffering with a stone, but will leave this to be done by practitioners of this work.

Into whatever houses I enter, I will go into them for the benefit of the sick and will abstain from every voluntary act of mischief and corruption; and, further, from the seduction of females or males, bond or free.

Whatever, in connection with my professional practice or not in connection with it, I may see or hear in the lives of men which ought not to be spoken of abroad, I will not divulge, reckoning that all such should be kept secret.

While I continue to keep this oath inviolate, may it be granted to me to enjoy life and the practice of the Art, respected by all men in all times, but should I trespass and violate this oath, may the reverse be my lot.

Notes

Chapter 1: Could It Be a Stealth Infection?

4–5 seborrheic dermatitis

Schwartz RA, Janusz CA, Janniger CK. Seborrheic dermatitis: an overview. *American Family Physician*. 2006; 74: 125–30.

5 cytomegalovirus is a member of the herpesvirus family

Taylor GH. Cytomegalovirus. *American Family Physician*. 2003; 67: 519–23.

6 bacterial overgrowth of the small intestine

Pimentel M, Chow EJ, Lin, HC. Eradication of small intestinal bacterial overgrowth reduces symptoms of irritable bowel syndrome. *American Journal of Gastroenterology*. 2000; 95: 3503–6.

8 *Giardia* . . . for decades if not properly treated

Kucik CJ, Martin GL, Sortor BV. Common intestinal parasites. *American Family Physician*. 2004; 69: 1161–65.

9 treatment has been shown to be effective

Ables AZ, Simon I, Melton ER. Update on *Helicobacter pylori* treatment. *American Family Physician*. 2007; 75: 351–54.

10 published in *American Medical News*

Landers SJ. Infection eyed as culprit in chronic disease. *American Medical News*. 2004; (July 19): 1–4.

Chapter 2: Normal Flora or Infection in the Body?

22 at the same time progressive dementia

Anderson M. Neurology of Whipple's disease. *Journal of Neurology, Neurosurgery, and Psychiatry*. 2000; 68: 2–5.

Verhagen WI, Huygen PL, Dalman JE, Schuurmans MM. Whipple's disease and the central nervous system. *Clinical Neurology and Neurosurgery*. 1996; 98: 299–304.

33 exposure to a varied group of microbes

von Mutius E. The increase in asthma can be ascribed to cleanliness.

American Journal of Respiratory and Critical Care Medicine. 2001; 164: 1106–7.

34   healthy body as opposed to one with disease

Blaser MJ. Who are we? Indigenous microbes and the ecology of human diseases. *European Molecular Biology Organization Reports.* 2006; 7: 956–60.

36   in causing cardiovascular and kidney diseases

Scannapieco FA. Position paper of The American Academy of Periodontology: periodontal disease as a potential risk factor for systemic diseases. *Journal of Periodontology.* 1998; 69: 841–50.

43   How do probiotics work?

Abramowicz M (editor). Probiotics. *The Medical Letter.* 2007; 49: 66–68.

47   Antiviral medications exist against fewer than a dozen of the thousands "Drugs for non-HIV viral infections". *The Medical Letter.* 2002; 44: 9–16.

Colgan R, Michocki R, Greisman L, Wolff Moore TA. Antiviral Drugs in the Immunocompetent Host. *American Family Physician,* 2003; 67: 757–67.

Chapter 3: How Medical Conditions and Stealth Germs Are Diagnosed

64   Expose the patient to a significant dose of radiation

Lockwood D, Einstein D, Davros W. Diagnostic imaging: radiation dose and patients' concerns. *Cleveland Clinic Journal of Medicine.* 2006; 73: 583–87.

Bui KL, Horner JD, Herts BR, Einstein DM. Intravenous iodinated contrast agents: risks and problematic situations. *Cleveland Clinic Journal of Medicine.* 2007; 74: 361–67.

Mitka M. MRI contrast agents may pose risk for patients with kidney disease. *Journal of the American Medical Association.* 2007; 297: 252–53.

67   interrupt the patient within the first half minute.

Barrier PA, Li JTC, Jensen, NM. Two words to improve physician-patient communication: what else? *Mayo Clinic Proceedings*. 2003. 78: 211–14.

Beckman HB, Frankel RM. The effect of physician behavior on the collection of data. *Annals of Internal Medicine*. 1984; 101: 692–96.

75   carrying certain other of the herpesviruses

Arvin A, Campadelli-Fiume G, et al. eds. *Human Herpesviruses: Biology, Therapy, and Immunoprophylaxis*. Cambridge University Press; 2007: 7-18.

See also International Herpes Management Forum at www.ihmf.org.

75   syphilis infection being the "great masquerader"

Brown DL, Frank JE. Diagnosis and management of syphilis. *American Family Physician*. 2003; 68: 297–305.

76–7 Nobel Prize was awarded to the Australian physicians

Parsonnet J. Clinician-discoverers—Marshall, Warren, and *H. pylori*. *New England Journal of Medicine*. 2005; 353: 2421–23.

78   Another danger of harboring a stealth infection

St. Georgiev V. *Infectious Diseases in Immunocompromised Hosts*. CRC Press 1998: 4-11.

78   so-called dual infection

Abu-Raddad LJ, Patnaik P, Kublin JG. Dual infection with HIV and malaria fuels the spread of both diseases in sub-Saharan Africa. *Science*. 2006; 314: 1603–6.

79   these days adhere to the principles of evidence-based medicine

Sackett DL, Rosenberg WM, Gray JA, Haynes RB, Richardson WS. Evidence based medicine: what it is and what it isn't. *British Medical Journal*. 1996: 312: 71–72.

Chapter 4: Stealth Infections of Body Regions

85   ulcer bacteria causing ulcers

Suerbaum S, Michetti P. *Helicobacter pylori* infection. *New England Journal of Medicine*. 2002; 347: 1175–86.

Ables AZ, Simon I, Melton ER. Update on *Helicobacter pylori* treatment. *American Family Physician*, 2007; 75: 351–57.

86   *Giardia lamblia*

Holtan NR. Giardiasis: a crimp in the life-style of campers, travelers, and others. *Postgraduate Medicine*. 1988; 83: 54–61.

Marshall MM, Naumovitz D, Ortega Y, Sterling CR. Waterborne protozoan pathogens. *Clinical Microbiology Reviews*. 1997; 10: 67–85.

87   Fitz-Hugh-Curtis syndrome

Peter NG, Clark LR, Jaeger JR. Fitz-Hugh-Curtis syndrome: a diagnosis to consider in women with right upper quadrant pain. *Cleveland Clinic Journal of Medicine*. 2004; 71: 233–39.

88   *Candida*

Weerasuriya N, Snape J. A study of *Candida esophagitis* in elderly patients attending a district general hospital in the UK. *Diseases of the Esophagus*. 2006: 19: 189–92.

89   arthirits and other symptoms caused by Lyme disease

Sigal LH. Myths and facts about Lyme disease. *Cleveland Clinic Journal of Medicine*. 1997: 64, 203–9.

Steere AC. Lyme disease. *New England Journal of Medicine*. 2001; 345: 115–25.

Depietropaolo DL, Powers JH, Gill JM. Diagnosis of Lyme disease. *American Family Physician*. 2005; 72: 297–304.

Hayes EB, Piesman J. How can we prevent Lyme disease? *New England Journal of Medicine*. 2003; 348: 2424–30.

Gayle A, Ringdahl E. Tick-borne diseases. *American Family Physician*. 2001; 64: 461–66.

89   Reiter's syndrome

Barth WF, Segal K. Reactive arthritis (Reiter's syndrome). *American Family Physician*. 1999: 60: 499–506.

90   rheumatoid arthritis

Tilley BC, Alarcón GS, Heyse SP, et al. Minocycline in rheumatoid arthritis. *Annals of Internal Medicine*. 1995; 122: 81–89.

91   arthritis due to gonorrhea

Rice PA. Gonococcal arthritis (disseminated gonococcal infection). *Infectious Disease Clinics of North America*. 2005; 19: 853–61.

Spadafora R. Case 19-2007: a college student with fever and joint pain. *New England Journal of Medicine*. 2007; 357: 1779–80.

Margaretten ME, Kholwes J, Moore D, Bent S. Does this adult patient have septic arthritis? *Journal of the American Medical Association*. 2007; 297: 1478–88.

92 reactivated infection with coccidioidomycosis

Wallis RS, Broder MS, Wong JY, Hanson ME, Beenhouwer DO. Granulomatous infectious diseases associated with tumor necrosis factor antagonists. *Clinical Infectious Diseases*. 2004; 38: 1261–65.

94 reactive arthritis caused by parvovirus B19

Martin DR, Schlott DW, Flynn JA. Clinical problem-solving. No respecter of age. *New England Journal of Medicine*. 2007; 357: 1856–59.

Kothari TH, Doshi DH. Managing human parvovirus B19-associated arthritis. *Journal of Musculoskeletal Medicine*. 2006; (December), 851–52.

96 syphilis, the "great masquerader"

Golden MR, Marra CM, Holmes KK. Update on syphilis: resurgence of an old problem. *Journal of the American Medical Association*. 2003; 290: 1510–14.

97 leukemia caused by viral infection

Murata K, Yamada Y. The state of the art in the pathogenesis of ATL and new potential targets associated with HTLV-1 and ATL. *International Reviews of Immunology*. 2007; 26: 249–68.

98 reactivation of malaria acquired abroad

Late relapse of *Plasmodium ovale* malaria. *Journal of the American Medical Association*. 2006; 295: 154–55.

99 cytomegalovirus

Aiello AE, Haan M, Blythe L, Moore K, Gonzalez JM, Jagust W. The influence of latent viral infection on rate of cognitive decline over 4 years. *Journal of the American Geriatrics Society*. 2006: 54: 1046–54.

Taylor GH. Cytomegalovirus. *American Family Physician*. 2003; 67: 519–24.

100 immune thrombocytopenic purpura

Emilia G, Luppi M, Zucchini P, et al. *Helicobacer pylori* infection and chronic immune thrombocytopenic purpura. *Blood*. 2007; 110: 3833–41.

101 blood transfusions transmitting various infections

Blajchman, MA, Vamvakas, EC. The continuing risk of transfusion-transmitted infections. *New England Journal of Medicine.* 2006; 355: 1303–5.

102 acquired pure red cell aplasia

Attar EC, Aquino SL, Hasserjian, RP. Case 33-2007: a 49-year-old HIV-positive man with anemia. *New England Journal of Medicine.* 2007; 357: 1745–54.

103 osteomyelitis caused by staphylococcus

Ptaszynski AE, Hooten WM, Huntoon MA. The incidence of spontaneous epidural abscess in Olmsted County from 1990 through 2000: a rare cause of spinal pain. *Pain Medicine.* 2007; 8: 338–43.

104 osteomyelitis from reactivated tuberculosis

Tuli SM. Tuberculosis of the spine: a historical review. *Clinical Orthopaedics and Related Research.* 2007; 460: 29–38.

105 irritable bowel syndrome due to *Giardia*

Kucik CJ, Martin GL, Sortor BV. Common intestinal parasites. *American Family Physician.* 2004; 69: 1161–68.

Sohail MR, Fischer P. *Blastocystis hominis* and travelers. *Travel Medicine and Infectious Disease.* 2005; 3: 33–38.

Arslan H, Inci EK, Azap OK, Karakayali H, Torgay A, Haberal M. Etiologic agents of diarrhea in solid organ recipients. *Transplant Infectious Disease.* 2007: 9: 270–75.

107 persistent diarrhea following antibiotic use

Sunenshine RH, McDonald LC. *Clostridium difficile*–associated disease: new challenges from an established pathogen. *Cleveland Clinic Journal of Medicine.* 2006; 73: 187–96.

108 Small intestine bacterial overgrowth

Schiller LR. Evaluation of small bowel bacterial overgrowth. *Current Gastroenterology Reports.* 2007; 9: 373–77.

108 Whipple's disease

Fenollar F, Puéchal X, Raoult D. Whipple's disease. *New England Journal of Medicine.* 2007; 356: 55–66.

109 inflammatory bowel disease

Hampton T. Scientists explore pathogenesis of IBD. *Journal of the American Medical Association.* 2004; 292: 2708–13.

Abraham C, Cho JH. Bugging of the intestinal mucosa. *New England Journal of Medicine.* 2007; 357: 708–10.

110 proctitis due to sexually transmitted diseases

Fried R, Surawicz C. Proctitis and sexually transmissible disease of the colon. *Current Treatment Options in Gastroenterology.* 2003; 6: 263–70.

110 salmonella carrier state

Roumagnac P, Weill FX, Dolecek C, et al. Evolutionary history of *Salmonella typhi. Science.* 2006; 314: 1301–4.

Xavier G. Management of typhoid and paratyphoid fevers. *Nursing Times.* 2006; 102: 49–51.

Falkow S. Is persistent bacterial infection good for your health? *Cell.* 2006; 124: 699–702.

112 dementia caused by neurosyphilis

Almeida OP, Lautenschlager NT. Dementia associated with infectious diseases. *International Psychogeriatrics.* 2005; 17 Suppl 1; S65–77.

Barrett AM. Is it Alzheimer's disease or something else? 10 disorders that may feature impaired memory and cognition. *Postgraduate Medicine.* 2005; 117: 47–53.

O'Donnell JA, Emery CL. Neurosyphilis: a current review. *Current Infectious Disease Reports.* 2005; 7: 277–84.

113 schizophrenia linked to exposure to certain infections

Jones J, Lopez A, Wilson M. Congenital toxoplasmosis. *American Family Physician.* 2003; 67; 2131–38.

Webster JP, Lamberton PH, Donnelly CA, Torrey EF. Parasites as causative agents of human affective disorders? *Proceedings: Biological Sciences.* 2006; 273: 1023–30.

Brown AS, Schaefer CA, Quesenberry CP Jr, Liu L, Babulas VP, Susser ES. Maternal exposure to toxoplasmosis and risk of schizophrenia in adult offspring. *American Journal of Psychiatry.* 2005; 162: 767–73.

Nellåker C, Yao Y, Jones-Brando L, Mallet F, Yolken RH, Karlsson

H. Transactivation of elements in the human endogenous retrovirus W family by viral infection. *Retrovirology*. 2006; 3: 44.

Kim JJ, Shirts BH, Dayal M, et al. Are exposure to cytomegalovirus and genetic variation on chromosome 6p joint risk factors for schizophrenia? *Annals of Medicine*. 2007; 39:145–53.

114 herpesvirus spreading to the brain

Tyler KL. Update on herpes simplex encephalitis. *Reviews in Neurological Diseases*. 2004; 1:169–78.

114 Dickerson FB, Boronow JJ, Stallings CR, Origoni AE, Yolken RH. Reduction of Symptoms by Valacyclovir in Cytomegalovirus— Seropositive Individuals With Schizophrenia. *American Journal of Psychiatry*. 2003; 160: 2234–6.

116 epilepsy linked to tropical infections

Kraft R. Cysticercosis: an emerging parasitic disease. *American Family Physician*. 2007; 76: 91–96.

117 Creutzfeldt-Jakob disease

Johnson RT, Gibbs CJ Jr. Creutzfeldt-Jakob disease and related transmissible spongiform encephalopathies. *New England Journal of Medicine*. 1998; 339: 1994–2004.

Geschwind MD, Haman A, Miller BL. Rapidly progressive dementia. *Neurologic Clinics*. 2007; 25: 783–807.

117 lymphocytic choriomeningitis virus

Fischer SA, Graham MB, Kuehnert MJ, et al. Transmission of lymphocytic choriomeningitis virus by organ transplantation. *New England Journal of Medicine*. 2006; 354: 2235–49.

Peters CJ. Lymphocytic choriomeningitis virus—an old enemy up to new tricks. *New England Journal of Medicine*. 2006; 354: 2208–11.

118 breast cancer in some cases

Melana SM, Nepomnaschy I, Sakalian M, Abbott A, Hasa J, Holland JF, Pogo BG. Characterization of viral particles isolated from primary cultures of human breast cancer cells. *Cancer Research*. 2007; 67: 8960–65.

119 cancer of the cervix in women

Schiffman M, Castle PE, Jeronimo J, Rodriguez AC, Wacholder S.

Human papillomavirus and cervical cancer. *Lancet*. 2007; 370: 890–907.

120 cancer of the liver caused by hepatitis

Marrero CR, Marrero JA.Viral hepatitis and hepatocellular carcinoma. *Archives of Medical Research*. 2007; 38: 612–20.

121 cancer of the lymph nodes

Brady G, MacArthur GJ, Farrell, PJ. Epstein-Barr virus and Burkitt lymphoma. *Journal of Clinical Pathology*. 2007; 60: 1397–1402.

Rezk SA, Weiss LM. Epstein-Barr virus–associated lymphoproliferative disorders. *Human Pathology*. 2007; 38: 1293–304.

121 sarcoma, a rare form of cancer

Antman K, Chang Y. Kaposi's sarcoma. *New England Journal of Medicine*. 2000; 342: 1027–38.

122 stomach cancer linked to ulcer bacteria

Correa P. Houghton J. Carcinogenesis of *Helicobacter pylori*. *Gastroenterology*. 2007; 133: 659–72.

123 Hodgkin's disease linked to cytomegalovirus

Huang G, Yan Q, Wang Z, Chen X, Zhang X, Guo Y, Li JJ. Human cytomegalovirus in neoplastic cells of Epstein-Barr virus negative Hodgkin's disease. *International Journal of Oncology*. 2002; 21: 31–36.

Toy JL, Knowlden RP. Cytomegalovirus retinitis misdiagnosed as Hodgkin's lymphoma deposits. *British Medical Journal*. 1978; 2: 1398–99.

124 cholangiocarcinoma caused by liver flukes

Schwartz DA. Cholangiocarcinoma associated with liver fluke infection: a preventable source of morbidity in Asian immigrants. *American Journal of Gastroenterology*. 1986; 81: 76–79.

125 squamous cancer of the bladder

Ross AG, Bartley PB, Sleigh AC, et al. Schistosomiasis. *New England Journal of Medicine*. 2002; 346: 1212–20.

125 sudden hearing loss may be

Rabinstein A, Jerry J, Saraf-Lavi E, Sklar E, Bradley WG. Sudden sensorineural hearing loss associated with herpes simplex virus type 1 infection. *Neurology*. 2001; 56: 571–72.

Gross M, Wolf DG, Elidan J, Eliashar R. Enterovirus, cytomegalovirus, and Epstein-Barr virus infection screening in idiopathic sudden sensorineural hearing loss. *Audiology and Neurotology*. 2007; 12: 179–82.

126 vertigo due to viral labyrinthitis

Ergul Y, Ekici B, Tastan Y, Sezer T, Uysal S. Vestibular neuritis caused by enteroviral infection. *Pediatric Neurology*. 2006; 34: 45–46.

128 virus may trigger childhood diabetes

Peng H, Hagopian W. Environmental factors in the development of Type 1 diabetes. *Reviews in Endocrine and Metabolic Disorders*. 2006: 7: 149–62.

van der Werf N, Kroese FG, Rozing J, Hillebrands JL. Viral infections as potential triggers of Type 1 diabetes. *Diabetes/Metabolism Research and Reviews*. 2007; 23: 169–83.

129 inflammation of the thyroid

Bach JF. Infections and autoimmune diseases. *Journal of Autoimmunity*. 2005; 25 Suppl: 74–80.

130 adrenal insufficiency (Addison's disease) due to

Haddara WM, van Uum SH. TB and adrenal insufficiency (letter). *Canadian Medical Association Journal*. 2004; 171: 710.

Carey RM. The changing clinical spectrum of adrenal insufficiency. *Annals of Internal Medicine*. 1997; 127: 1102–5.

132 episodic burning in the esophagus

McKenna DP, Triner W, Tomassi M, Poonthota A. Herpes simplex virus esophagitis in an immunocompetent teenaged girl. *American Journal of Emergency Medicine*. 2006; 24: 902–4.

133 chronically irritated eyelids due to rosacea

Stone DU, Chodosh J. Ocular rosacea: an update on pathogenesis and therapy. *Current Opinion in Opthalmology*. 2004; 15: 499–502.

134 rapidly progressive inflammation in the eye

Balansard B, Bodaghi B, Cassoux N, et al. Necrotising retinopathies simulating acute retinal necrosis syndrome. *British Journal of Ophthalmology*, 2005; 89: 96–101.

135 pain in eye followed by

Shaikh S, Ta CN. Evaluation and management of herpes zoster ophthalmicus. *American Family Physician*. 2002; 66: 1723–30.

136 chronic fatigue syndrome (CFS)

Craig T, Kakumanu S. Chronic fatigue syndrome: evaluation and treatment. *American Family Physician*. 2002; 65: 1083–90.

Jason LA, Fennell PA, Taylor RR, eds. *Handbook of Chronic Fatigue Syndrome*. John Wiley & Sons, 2003: 38-49.

Evengård B, Klimas N. Chronic fatigue syndrome: probable pathogenesis and possible treatments. *Drugs*. 2002; 62: 2433–46.

Hampton T. Chronic fatigue answers sought. *Journal of the American Medical Association*. 2006; 296: 2915.

136 Gulf War syndrome are puzzing conditions

Sartin JS. Gulf War syndrome: the final chapter? *Mayo Clinic Proceedings*. 2006; 81: 1425–26.

137 Lyme disease

Sigal LH. Myths and facts about Lyme disease. *Cleveland Clinic Journal of Medicine*, 1997: 64, 203–9. Steere AC. Lyme disease. *New England Journal of Medicine*. 2001; 345: 115–19.

DePietropaolo DL, Powers JH, Gill JM, Foy AJ. Diagnosis of Lyme disease. *American Family Physician*. 2005; 72: 297–304.

138 hepatitis B or C

Lee, WM. Hepatitis B virus infection. *New England Journal of Medicine*. 1997; 337: 1733–45.

Lauer GM, Walker BD. Hepatitis C virus infection. *New England Journal of Medicine*. 2001; 345: 41–52.

139 chronic fatigue syndrome attributed in some to Mycoplasma

Nicolson GL, Gan R, Haier J. Multiple co-infections (Mycoplasma, Chlamydia, human herpes virus-6) in chronic fatigue syndrome patients: association with signs and symptoms. *Acta Pathologica, Microbiologica, et Immunologica Scandinavica*. 2003; 111: 557—66.

140 Poorly healing sores around the ankles.

Noble SL, Forbes RC, Stamm PL. Diagnosis and management of common tinea infections, *American Family Physician*. 1998; 58: 163–74.

141 Gynecologic and pelvic conditions.

McCormack WM. Pelvic inflammatory disease. *New England Journal of Medicine*. 1994: 330, 115–19.

Bossard S, Knapp B. When to suspect pelvic inflammatory disease. *Emergency Medicine*. 2004; 36: 45–50.

Peter NG, Clark LR, Jaeger JR. Fitz-Hugh-Curtis syndrome: a diagnosis to consider in women with right upper quadrant pain. *Cleveland Clinic Journal of Medicine*. 2004; 71, 233–39.

Owen MK, Clenney TL. Management of vaginitis. *American Family Physician*. 2004; 70: 2125–32.

Anderson MR, Klink K, Cohrssen A. Evaluation of vaginal complaints. *Journal of the American Medical Association*, 2004; 291: 1368–79.

144 chronic sinus infection causing malaise

Rice DH. Clearing up chronic rhinosinusitis: practical steps to take. *Journal of Respiratory Diseases*. 2005; 26: 415–22.

146 heart and cardiovascular conditions

Kuppuswamy VC, Gupta S. Antibiotic therapy for coronary heart disease: the myth and the reality. *Timely Topics in Medicine: Cardiovascular Diseases*. 2006; 10, E2.

Ellis CR, Di Salvo T. Myocarditis: basic and clinical aspects. *Cardiology Reviews*. 2007; 15: 170–7.

Feldman AM, McNamara D. Myocarditis. *New England Journal of Medicine*. 2000; 343: 1388–98.

Franco-Paredes C, Rouphael N, Méndez J, et al. Cardiac manifestations of parasitic infections. Part 2: Parasitic myocardial disease. *Cinical Cardiology*. 2007; 30: 218–22.

Kytö V, Vuorinen T, Saukko P, et al. Cytomegalovirus infection of the heart is common in patients with fatal myocarditis. *Clinical Infectious Diseases*. 2005; 40: 683–8.

Paterick TE, Paterick TJ, Nishimura RA, Steckelberg JM. Complexity and subtlety of infective endocarditis. *Mayo Clinic Proceedings*. 2007; 82: 615—21.

Mylonakis E. Calderwood SB. Infective endocarditis in adults. *New

England Journal of Medicine. 2001; 354: 1318–29.

Pagnoux C, Cohen P, Guillevin L. Vasculitides secondary to infections. *Clinical and Experimental Rheumatology.* 2006; 24 (2 Suppl 41): S71–81.

150 kidneys and stealth infections

Hricik DE, Chung-Park M. Sedor, JR. Glomerulonephritis. *New England Journal of Medicine.* 1998; 339: 888–99.

Wen MC, Lian JD, Chang HR, et al. Polyomavirus nephropathy in renal allograft: prevalence and correlation of histology with graft failure. *Nephrology.* 2007; 12: 615–19.

Maddirala S, Pitha JV, Cowley BD Jr, Haragsim L. End-stage renal disease due to polyomavirus in a cardiac transplant patient. *Nature Clinical Practice: Nephrology.* 2007; 3: 393–96.

154 spots on the liver on X-ray

Kurowski R, Ostapchuk M. Overview of histoplasmosis. *American Family Physician.* 2002; 66: 2247–52.

Chandra D, Manikdiyil BJ, Guy E, Hamill RJ. Latent Enigma. *American Journal of Medicine.* 2006; 119: 581–83.{}

155 chronic bronchitis nonresponsive to

Bhadriraju S, Cooper KR. Pulmonary infections with MAC: diagnosis and management. *Journal of Respiratory Diseases.* 2003; 24: 127–135.

Pérez-Yarza EG, Moreno A, Lázaro P, Mejías A, Ramilo O. The association between respiratory syncytial virus infection and the development of childhood asthma: a systematic review of the literature. *Pediatric Infectious Disease Journal.* 2007; 26: 733–39.

Bisgaard H, Hermansen MN, Buchvald F, et al. Childhood asthma after bacterial colonization of the airway in neonates. *New England Journal of Medicine.* 2007; 357: 1487–95.

Knutsen AP. Untreated ABPA can cause irreversible lung damage: when to suspect allergic bronchopulmonary aspergillosis. *Journal of Respiratory Diseases.* 2006; 27: 123–34.

Jasmer RM, Nahid P, Hopewell PC. Clinical Practice: latent tuberculosis infection. *New England Journal of Medicine.* 2002; 347: 1860–66.

159 chronic prostatitis in men

Potts J, Payne RE. Prostatitis: infection, neuromuscular disorder, or pain syndrome? *Cleveland Clinic Journal of Medicine.* 2007; 74 (Suppl): S63–71.

160   prostate cancer rarely

Sarma AV, McLaughlin JC, Wallner LP, et als. Sexual behavior, sexually transmitted diseases and prostatitis: the risk of prostate cancer in black men. *Journal of Urology.* 2006; 176: 1108–13.

Dong B, Kim S, Hong S, et al. An infectious retrovirus susceptible to an IFN antiviral pathway from human prostate tumors. *Proceedings of the National Academy of Sciences.* 2007; 104: 1655-60.

Mackay IM, Harnett G, Jeoffreys N, et al. Detection and discrimination of herpes simplex viruses, *Haemophilus ducreyi, Treponema pallidum,* and *Calymmatobacterium (Klebsiella) granulomatis* from genital ulcers. *Clinical Infectious Diseases.* 2006; 42: 1431–38.

165   mouth and throat

Gonsalves WC, Chi AC, Neville BW. Common oral lesions: Part 1. Superficial mucosal lesions. *American Family Physician.* 2007; 75: 501–7.

Ali AA, Suresh CS. Oral lichen planus in relation to transaminase levels and hepatitis C virus. *Journal of Oral Patholgy and Medicine.* 2007; 36: 604–8.

167   trichinosis from pork

Pozio E, Darwin Murrell K. Systematics and epidemiology of trichinella. *Advances in Parasitology.* 2006; 63: 367–439.

Most H. Trichinosis—preventable yet still with us. *New England Journal of Medicine.* 1978; 298: 1178–80.

168   multiple sclerosis

Krone B, Pohl D. Rostasy K, et al. Common infectious agents in multiple sclerosis: a case-control study in children. *Multiple Sclerosis.* 2007; 14: 136–39.

Lipton HL, Liang Z, Hertzler S, Son KN. A specific viral cause of multiple sclerosis: one virus, one disease. *Annals of Neurology.* 2007; 61: 514–23.

Lünemann JD, Münz C. Epstein-Barr virus and multiple sclerosis.

Current Neurology and Neuroscience Reports. 2007; 7: 253–58.

Hughes RA, Cornblath DR. Guillain-Barré syndrome. *Lancet.* 2005; 366: 1653–66.

171 chronic irritation inside the lining of the nostrils

Dall'Antonia M, Coen PG, Wilks M. Whiley A. Millar M. Competition between methicillin-sensitive and -resistant *Staphylococcus aureus* in the anterior nares. *Journal of Hospital Infection.* 2005; 61: 62–67.

Riechelmann H, Essig A, Deutschle T. Rau A, Rothermel B, Weschta M. Nasal carriage of *Staphylococcus aureus* in house dust mite allergic patients and healthy controls. *Allergy.* 2005; 60: 1418–23.

174 obesity and stealth germs

Atkinson RL. Viruses as an etiology of obesity. *Mayo Clinic Proceedings.* 2007; 82: 1192–98.

Turnbaugh PJ, Ley RE, Mahowald MA, Magrini V, Mardis ER, Gordon JI. An obesity-associated gut microbiome with increased capacity for energy harvest. *Nature.* 2006; 444: 1027–31.

Dhurandhar NV, Kulkarni PR, Ajinkya SM, Sherikar AA, Atkinson RL. Association of adenovirus infection with human obesity. *Obesity Research.* 1997: 5: 464–69.

176 stealth infections and the skin

Schwartz RA, Nervi SJ. Erythema nodosum: a sign of systemic disease. *American Family Physician.* 2007; 75: 695–700.

177 seborrheic dermatitis

Schwartz RA, Janusz CA, Janniger CK. Seborrheic dermatitis: an overview. *American Family Physician.* 2006; 74: 125–30.

178 rosacea

Powell FC. Clinical practice: rosacea. *New England Journal of Medicine.* 2005; 352: 793–803.

179 viruses and skin cancer

Molho-Pessach V, Lotem, M. Viral carcinogenesis in skin cancer. *Current Problems in Dermatology.* 2007; 35: 39–51.

179 hives occasionally associated with underlying sinus infection

Gershwin EM, Watson, RD. Clinical consultation: is there a connection between urticaria and sinusitis? *Journal of Respiratory Diseases.*

2002; 23, 214.

Suzuki H, Marshall BJ, Hibi T. Overview: *Helicobacter pylori* and extragastric disease. *International Journal of Hematology*. 2006; 84: 291–300.

Gupta R, Parsi K. Chronic urticaria due to *Blastocystis hominis*. *Australasian Journal of Dermatology*. 2006; 47: 117–19.

Singla R, Brodell RT. Erythema multiforme due to herpes simplex virus. *Postgraduate Medicine*. 1999; 106: 151–53.

183 interstitial cystitis

Fioriti D, Penta M, Mischitelli M, et al. Interstitial cystitis and infectious agents. *International Journal of Immunopathology and Pharmacology*. 2005; 18: 799–804.

Atug F, Turkeri L, Atug O, Cal C. Detection of *Helicobacter pylori* in bladder biopsy specimens of patients with interstitial cystitis by polymerase chain reaction. *Urological Research*. 2004; 32: 346–49.

Chapter 5: Special Conditions

187 and to textbooks of perinatology, obstetrics, and infectious diseases.

Kirkham C, Harris S, Grzybowski S. Evidence-based prenatal care: part II, third-trimester care and prevention of infectious diseases. *American Family Physician*. 2005; 71: 1555–60.

Also see Infections During Pregnancy on www.perinatology.com.

188 pregnant women with the staph organism

Chen KT, Huard RC, Della-Latta P, Saiman L. Prevalence of methicillin-sensitive and methicillin-resistant *Staphylococcus aureus* in pregnant women. *Obsetrics and Gynecology*. 2006; 108: 482–87.

188 parvovirus B19

Servey JT, Reamy BV, Hodge J. Clinical presentations of parvovirus B19 infection. *American Family Physician*. 2007; 75: 373–76.

189 making motherhood safe in developing countries

Rosenfield A, Min CJ, Freedman LP. Making Motherhood Safe in Developing Countries. *New England Journal of Medicine*. 2007; 356: 1395–97.

191 can they also be the source of potentially hazardous infections

Morrison G. Zoonotic infections from pets: understanding the risks and treatment. *Postgraduate Medicine.* 2001; 110: 24–36.

Rabinowitz PM, Gordon Z, Odofin L. Pet-related Infections. *American Family Physician.* 2007; 76: 1314–22.

Kuehn BM. Antibiotic-resistant "superbugs" may be transmitted from animals to humans. *Journal of the American Medical Association.* 2007; 298: 2125–26.

Gayle A, Ringdahl E. Tick-borne diseases. *American Family Physician.* 2001; 64: 461–66.

Kuehn BM. Animal-human diseases targeted to stop pandemics before they start. *Journal of the American Medical Association.* 2006; 295, 1987–89.

Kahn LH, Kaplan B, Monath TP, Steele JH. Teaching "one medicine, one health." *The American Journal of Medicine.* 2008; 121:169-70.

Chapter 6: What Else Could It Be?

197 some of the treatable viruses are

Colgan R, Michocki R, Greisman L, Moore TA. Antiviral drugs in the immunocompetent host: part 1, treatment of hepatitis, cytomegalovirus, and herpes infections. *American Family Physician.* 2003; 67: 757–62.

199 serum protein electrophoresis

O'Connell TX, Horita TJ, Kasravi B. Understanding and interpreting serum protein electrophoresis. *American Family Physician.* 2005; 71: 105–10.

200 erythrocyte sedimentation rate

Bridgen, ML. Clinical utility of the erythrocyte sedimentation rate. *American Family Physician.* 1999; 60: 1443–50.

209 caused by household mold and candida

Khalili B, Montanaro MT, Bardana EJ Jr. Indoor mold and your patient's health: from suspicion to confirmation. *Journal of Respiratory Diseases.* 2005; 26: 520–25.

Kuhn DM, Ghannoum MA. Indoor mold, toxigenic fungi, and Stachybotrys charatrum: infectious disease perspective. *Clinical*

Microbiology Reviews, 2003; 16: 144–72.

211   relationship between damp buildings and

Tomaselli KP. How to treat a sick office: go after hidden environmental factors. *American Medical News*. 2006; (December 18): 22–23.

212   it is extremely rare for it to spread in the form of

Rondon-Berrios H, Khilnani N, Trevejo-Nunez GJ. Disseminated candidiasis in intravenous drug abusers: a distinctive syndrome. *Johns Hopkins Advanced Studies in Medicine*. 2006; 6: 191–94.

214   are caused by fungal organisms whose spores are inhaled

Zaas AK, Perfect JR. Pulmonary fungal infections: making the diagnosis. *Journal of Respiratory Diseases*. 2003; 24, 433–44.

215   in persons receiving chemotherapy or medicines that suppress

Wallis RS, Broder MS, Wong JY, Hanson ME, Beenhouwer DO. Granulomatous infectious diseases associated with tumor necrosis factor antagonists. *Clinical Infectious Diseases*, 2004; 38: 1261–65.

218   damage from such an infection can predispose a person to have minimal, mild, moderate, or perhaps severe brain problems

Power C, Johnson RT, eds. *Emerging Neurological Infections*. Informa Healthcare, 2005.

Levenson JL. Psychiatric issues in infectious diseases. *Primary Psychiatry*. 2006; 13: 29–32.

225   an example of the complexities of treatment decisions

Elliott VS. Antibiotics ineffective in preventing heart attacks. *American Medical News*. 2004; (October 4), 32–33.

Cannon CP, Braunwald E, McCabe CH, et al. Antibiotic treatment of *Chlamydia pneumoniae* after acute coronary syndrome. *New England Journal of Medicine*, 2005; 352: 1646–54.

Chapter 7: Treatment Expectations

227   hepatitis C, treatment decisions are even more complicated.

Ward RP, Kugelmas M, Libsch K. Management of hepatitis C: evaluating suitability for drug therapy. *American Family Physician*. 2004; 69: 1429–36.

Hoofnagle JH, Seeff LB. Peginterferon and ribavirin for chronic hepatitis C. *New England Journal of Medicine.* 2006; 355: 2444–51.

228 CFS may be an infectious or post-infectious condition.

Craig T, Kakumanu S. Chronic fatigue syndrome: evaluation and treatment. *American Family Physician.* 2002; 65: 1083–90.

Jason LA, Fennell PA, Taylor RR, eds. *Handbook of Chronic Fatigue Syndrome.* John Wiley & Sons, 2003.

Evengård B, Klimas N. Chronic fatigue syndrome: probable pathogenesis and possible treatments. *Drugs.* 2002; 62: 2433–46.

Hampton T. Chronic fatigue answers sought. *Journal of the American Medical Association,* 2006; 296: 2915.

230 Gulf War syndrome is another well-known

Sartin JS. Gulf War syndrome: the final chapter? *Mayo Clinic Proceedings.* 2006; 81: 1425–26.

230 handful of cases of leishmaniasis

Markle WH, Makhoul K. Cutaneous leishmaniasis: recognition and treatment. *American Family Physician.* 2004; 69: 1455–60.

237 probiotics are not members of the normal flora of the body

Margolis S (editor). Stirring up helpful bacteria. *The Johns Hopkins Medical Letter (Health After 50).* 2002;14:1–7.

238 *Bifidobacterium infantis* helps improve the symptoms

Whorwell PJ, Altringer L, Morel J, Bond Y, et al. Efficacy of encapsulated probiotic *Bifidobacterium infantis* 35624 in women with irritable bowel syndrome. *American Journal of Gastroenterology.* 2006; 101: 1581–90.

Abramowicz M (editor). Probiotics. *The Medical Letter.* 2007; 49: 66–68.

240 preparation of these eggs has been reported to reduce disease activity

Reddy A, Fried B. The use of *Trichuris suis* and other helminth therapies to treat Crohn's Disease. *Parasitology Research.* 2007; 100: 921–27.

Chapter 8: Prevention

245 in the midst of a war with the microbial world, a resilient foe

Fauci AS. Emerging infectious diseases: a clear and present danger to humanity. *Journal of the American Medical Association.* 2004; 292: 1887–88.

248 health-care agencies promote prudent principles of hand-hygiene.
Mindell B. The first defense: soap and water. *American Medical News.*
2005 (November 28): 29.

Peterson LR, Singh K, Universal patient disinfection as a tool for
infection control. *Archives of Internal Medicine.* 2006; 166; 274–76.

D'Souza AL, Rajkumar C, Cooke J, Bulpitt CJ. Probiotics in prevention of antibiotic associated diarrhoea: meta-analysis. *British Medical
Journal.* 2002; 2: 1361.

Hickson M. D'Souza AL, Muthu N, et al. Use of probiotic
Lactobacillus preparation to prevent diarrhoea associated with
antibitocs. *British Medical Journal.* 2007; 335(7610): 80.

255 vaccinating against cancer is a remarkable new milestone
Fischman J. The World's First Cancer Vaccines: Sticking it to Cancer.
US News and World Report. 2006 (April 3): 56–63.

Ada G. Vaccines and vaccination. *New England Journal of Medicine.*
2001; 345: 1042–53.

Allen A. *Vaccine: The Controversial Story of Medicine's Greatest Lifesaver.*
New York: W. W. Norton, 2007.

Kimberlin DW, Whitley RJ. *Varicella-zoster* vaccine for the prevention of herpes zoster. *New England Journal of Medicine.* 2007; 356:
1338–43.

Steinbrook R. The potential of human papillomavirus vaccines. *New
England Journal of Medicine.* 2006; 354: 1109–12.

258 some persons are concerned that vaccines
Kimmel S. Vaccine adverse events: separating myth from reality.
American Family Physician. 2002; 66: 2113–20.

Acknowledgments

I owe many, many thanks to those who helped make this book a reality.

I am most grateful to Mollie Glick, my agent, of the Jean Naggar Literary Agency in New York, who had faith in my writing, sensed my passion for the topic, and helped bring this project to fruition. Special thanks to Patricia Gift at Sterling Publishing in New York, who accepted *Stealth Germs in Your Body* for publication, and to Philip Turner and his staff at Sterling, who helped bring it to completion.

I owe foremost thanks to my wife, Martha Peaslee Daniel, for her unfailing patience and understanding for my medical work, writing, and teaching activities over the years. She helped me greatly with this book, my newspaper columns, and other writings. Many thanks to my son, Mike (Michael P.) Daniel, who helped me with design and Web site details. I am also grateful to all of my family, who were patient with me during the time I wrote the book.

I wish to thank Tom English and Rebecca Springer for their thorough reading and editing of the manuscript and very useful recommendations. I am grateful for the help and work of project editor Rebecca Maines, and designer Chrissy Kwasnik. Many thanks also to Sara Miller McCune of Sage Publications, who made many helpful suggestions. I owe much to writers Susan and Everett Murdock, who helped immensely with writing details, and encouraged me. I am also grateful to Claire Earley, and my staff, who enthusiastically supported the project and helped me with patient care at Sansum Clinic while I was writing the book.

Thank you all! It is my hope that this book will be one small step toward improving the health of my fellow human beings.

Index

Note: Page numbers in *italics* indicate references to tables.